Promoting Physical Activity and Fitness

Supporting Individuals with Childhood-Onset Disabilities

T0312741

Promoting Physical Activity and Fitness

Supporting Individuals with Childhood-Onset Disabilities

Edited by

Désirée B Maltais

Associate Professor, Department of Rehabilitation, Université Laval, Quebec City, Canada; Researcher, Centre for Interdisciplinary Research in Rehabilitation and Social Integration, Quebec City, Canada

Reidun B Jahnsen

Head of the Research Department, Beitostølen Healthsports Centre, Beitostølen, Norway; Professor Emerita, Research Centre of Habilitation and Rehabilitation Models and Services (CHARM), Institute of Health and Society, University of Oslo, Oslo, Norway; Senior Researcher, Norwegian Quality and Surveillance Registry of Cerebral Palsy (NorCP), Oslo University Hospital, Oslo, Norway

2023
Mac Keith Press

Chief Executive: Ann-Marie Halligan
Senior Publishing Manager: Sally Wilkinson
Editorial and Marketing Co-ordinator: Polly Galis
Production Manager: Andy Booth

First published in this edition in 2023 by Mac Keith Press
2nd Floor, Rankin Building, 139–143 Bermondsey Street, London, SE1 3UW

British Library Cataloguing-in-Publication data
A catalogue record for this book is available from the British Library

Cover designer: Marten Sealby
Cover photograph credits: Beitostølen Healthsports Centre for the group and children in the pool photographs, and Thor Østbye/Beitostølen Healthsports Centre for the bike photograph.

ISBN: 978-1-911612-12-4
Typeset by Riverside Publishing Solutions Ltd
Printed by Hobbs the Printers Ltd, Totton, Hampshire, UK

Contents

Contents

Author Appointments

John Cairney
Professor and Head of School of Human Movement and Nutrition Sciences, University of Queensland, Brisbane, Australia.

Craig Campbell
Professor, Paediatrics, Clinical Neurological Sciences and Epidemiology, University of Western Ontario, London, Canada; Head Paediatric Neurology, Children's Hospital LHSC, London, Canada; Scientist, Children's Health Research Institute, London, Canada.

Haakon Dalen
Medical Doctor, Head of the Rehabilitation Department, Beitostølen Healthsports Center, Beitostølen, Norway.

Anne-Stine Dolva
Professor, Inland Norway University of Applied Sciences, Lillehammer, Norway.

Dot Dumuid
Senior Research Fellow, Alliance for Research in Exercise, Nutrition and Activity, University of South Australia, Adelaide, Australia.

Maria Terese Engdahl-Høgåsen
Freelance Dance Artist, Creator, and Teacher, Oslo, Norway.

Kaja Giltvedt
Physiotherapist, Frambu Resource Centre for Rare Disorders, Siggerud, Norway.

Berit Gjessing
Physiotherapist, Team Leader, Beitostølen Healthsports Centre, Beitostølen, Norway; PhD Candidate, University of Oslo, Institute of Health and Society, Oslo, Norway.

Jeffrey D Graham
Postdoctoral Fellow, Infant Child and Youth Health Lab, Child and Youth Studies, Brock University, St Catharines, Canada.

Erik H Hulzebos
ACSM Registered Clinical Exercise Physiologist and Sports Physical Therapist, Child Development and Exercise Center, University Medical Center, Utrecht, the Netherlands.

Reidun B Jahnsen
Head of the Research Department, Beitostølen Healthsports Centre, Beitostølen, Norway; Professor Emerita, Research Centre of Habilitation and Rehabilitation Models and Services (CHARM), Institute of Health and Society, University of Oslo, Oslo, Norway; Senior Researcher, Norwegian Quality and Surveillance Registry of Cerebral Palsy (NorCP), Oslo University Hospital, Oslo, Norway.

Sara King-Dowling
Research Associate, Section on Behavioral Oncology, Division of Oncology, The Children's Hospital of Philadelphia, Philadelphia, USA; Affiliated Scientist, Infant Child and Youth Health Lab, Child and Youth Studies, Brock University, St Catharines, Canada.

Carol Maher
Professor of Population and Digital Health, University of South Australia, Adelaide, Australia.

Désirée B Maltais
Associate Professor, Department of Rehabilitation, Université Laval, Quebec City, Canada; Researcher, Centre for Interdisciplinary Research in Rehabilitation and Social Integration, Quebec City, Canada.

Shubhra Mukherjee
Adjunct-Assistant Professor, Department of Physical Medicine and Rehabilitation, Feinberg School of Medicine, Northwestern University, Chicago, USA; Physiatrist, Shriners Children's Chicago, Chicago, USA.

Ellen K Munkhaugen
Unit Leader and Researcher, Norwegian National Advisory Unit on Mental Health in Intellectual Disabilities, Oslo University Hospital, Oslo, Norway.

Anne Ottestad
Engineer and Voluntary Sports Instructor, Friskis & Svettis, Bærum, Norway; Founder and Leader of *Upturn* and Mother of Kjersti Syvertsen.

Kristine Risum
Physiotherapist, Section for Orthopaedic Rehabilitation, Oslo University Hospital, Oslo, Norway; Physiotherapist, Norwegian National Advisory Unit of Rheumatic Diseases in Children and Adolescents, Section for Rheumatology, Oslo University Hospital, Oslo, Norway; Associate

Professor, Department of Rehabilitation Science and Health Technology, Faculty of Health Sciences, Oslo Metropolitan University, Oslo, Norway.

Ana-Marie Rojas
Assistant Professor of Physical Medicine and Rehabilitation, Feinberg School of Medicine, Northwestern University, Chicago, USA; Attending Physician, Shirley Ryan Ability Lab, Chicago, USA.

Andreas T Sandfossen
General Manager, Physiotherapy Institute, Solheimsvcien, Lørenskog, Norway.

Kjersti Syvertsen
Social Worker and Voluntary Sports Instructor, Friskis & Svettis, Bærum, Norway; Participant in *Upturn*.

Tim Takken
Associate Professor, Child Development and Exercise Center, Wilhelmina Children's Hospital, UMC Utrecht, Utrecht, the Netherlands.

Roald Undlien
Associate Professor, Inland Norway University of Applied Sciences, Lillehammer, Norway.

Katy de Valle
Senior Clinician and Researcher, Neurology Department, The Royal Children's Hospital, Melbourne, Australia; Research Assistant, Clinical Sciences, Neuroscience, Murdoch Children's Research Institute, Melbourne, Australia.

Olaf Verschuren
Assistant Professor, UMC Utrecht Brain Center and Center of Excellence for Rehabilitation Medicine, Utrecht University, Utrecht, the Netherlands.

Ine Wigernaes
Pro-rector for Public Relations, Department of Public Relations, Campus Lillehammer, Inland Norway University of Applied Sciences, Lillehammer, Norway.

Foreword

Exercise and physical activity in all forms are an important part of life for people with childhood-onset disabilities. They provide energy, help with the development and maintenance of physical and mental health and functional skills, and provide opportunity for the best possible quality of life. It is the same for me. I have unilateral (left-sided) spastic cerebral palsy and exercise has been and is a crucial part of my childhood and adult life.

Exercise for me includes running, going to the gym, playing ball sports, and judo. Because I enjoy training, my physical abilities develop in the best way, which contributes to the good quality of life I have today and hopefully will be able to maintain throughout my life. Keeping going and motivating yourself to continue training throughout life isn't always easy, but it is crucial to have the best quality of life and functional ability. I have witnessed this first-hand in my work as a physiotherapist and in my own physical training. It is important to have people around you who know you, your disability, and your physical abilities well, that you trust and who can motivate you to continue training and push yourself a little harder during sessions. Having good support from coaches and others motivated me and pushed me from being able to run 600m to running 10km in 57 minutes 30 seconds over 2 years. By starting slowly and by gradually increasing the time and speed of my runs, my fitness, strength, and body control improved.

If my trainer, those who supported me during that period, and I had access to the guidance in this book, we would have had better communication with each other. I would have been able to ask more questions, gain a better understanding of the training, and would have avoided some mistakes and setbacks. In addition, we could have found alternative ways to overcome obstacles, measure the training results, and get better results without compromising the safety of the exercises.

There is no doubt that people with disabilities can train hard, with many and long sessions according to their abilities. Based on my experience, I think it is good that we now have this book which contains useful information both for the persons with disabilities and for those who support them in their training, including how training sessions should best be laid out now and in the future.

The book focuses on describing fitness, strength, and flexibility training with physiological guidance. Comprehensive advice and information on healthy intensity, load, duration of training, and appropriate number of sessions per week is provided. Many examples of the tests used to measure the person's physical abilities are also given. The importance of individually adapting training according to the functional abilities of people with childhood-onset disabilities, their technical skills, age, and their abilities to follow instructions is made apparent. The authors explain the significance of good preparation, with useful tips and advice to consider for people with childhood-onset disabilities based on their specific disabilities. As many of these individuals may have pain, spasticity, epilepsy, vision and hearing impairments, and other difficulties described in the book, adaptations might be required to make exercise and activities safe. Chapter 3 gives specific advice on safety considerations, especially adapted to the needs of children and young people.

Measuring and understanding one's training progression is crucial for successful development, so the person with the disability and the trainer or the one who supports the physical activities can properly measure their effectiveness. Therefore, the book covers different measurement methods that are good to use, and how they can be combined for the best measurement results. There is a wide range of methods discussed, from advanced methods with laboratory analyses, to simpler methods, such as activity measurement through smart watches, diary writing, or self-assessment forms, with several other methods in between.

Being physically active and exercising is important for development and improves quality of life. Therefore, strategy and theory examples provided throughout the book will help people with childhood-onset disabilities, their trainer, or others who help with physical activities to stay motivated or make a behavioral change to ensure continued exercise throughout life. This can range from setting the right goals to increase self-esteem, to using activity-enhancing and technical aids as motivation for exercise.

In addition to guidance and advice that apply to anyone with childhood-onset disabilities, the book covers a lot of diagnosis-specific information for a wide variety of diagnoses including: cerebral palsy (Chapter 6), developmental coordination disorder (Chapter 7), spina bifida and childhood acquired spinal cord injury (Chapter 8), childhood-onset neuromuscular conditions (Chapter 9), intellectual disability (Chapter 10), autism spectrum disorder (Chapter 11), and juvenile idiopathic arthritis (Chapter 12).

Anyone with childhood-onset disabilities, their parents, trainers in sports associations, assistants, sports teachers, and others who take care of people with childhood-onset disabilities in training or movement contexts should read this book and have it by their side as a guide in all phases of training. Not only is it a good support for setting up adapted training at a suitable and challenging level in the present, but it also helps the reader find ways to keep training over time. It encourages measuring progress and enhances understanding of how the training works, to ensure it continues in an appropriate and safe way.

Linda Sandström
Research Assistant and Physiotherapist, Orthopedics,
Department of Clinical Sciences Lund, Lund University, Lund, Sweden.
Linda was born 3rd May 1991 and has unilateral cerebral palsy.

CHAPTER 1

Introduction

An Orientation to the Book and How to Use It

Désirée B Maltais and Reidun B Jahnsen

Being physically fit and active, as discussed in Chapters 2 and 4, respectively, can have lasting mental and physical health benefits if the person continues a lifestyle that promotes physical fitness and activity. Since people with childhood-onset disabilities are often less fit and active than their peers without a disability, promoting such a lifestyle over the long-term can be especially important to their overall health. However, present publications on the topic for the general population do not necessarily meet the specific needs of people with disabilities, and when such publications do consider these needs, they are often written for experts only or the information is incomplete within a given publication.

To address the issue, health and exercise science experts were tasked by the editors to provide the book's readers with physical fitness and activity information that is relevant to the childhood-onset disabilities covered in the book, which is based on scientific evidence and clinical experience, and can be understood by the general population of young people and adults, as well as professionals in the field. In this manner, the primary readers can be assured of having key information in one place.

The book's aim and its intended readers, main contents, and structure, as well as how one might use it, are described below.

WHAT IS THE AIM OF THE BOOK?

The book aims to empower people living with childhood-onset disabilities, and others who support them, to contribute to making informed decisions about fostering a lifestyle that promotes physical fitness and activity over the long-term.

WHO IS THE BOOK WRITTEN FOR?

The intended readers of the book are:

- People with childhood-onset disabilities;
- Their families and caregivers;
- People with a health or exercise science background;
- Health and exercise science students;
- Individuals in the community without a health or exercise science background who are supporting or wish to support the physical fitness and activity of this group.

In some cases, people with childhood-onset physical disabilities may find the book's contents difficult to understand due to their age, or due to reading or other difficulties. In these instances, the contents can be used by families, caregivers, and others to help inform the individual so they can nevertheless take part in decision-making.

People who wish to support the physical fitness and activity of this group who have a health or exercise science background, but not both, may find the book useful as a starting point for information they are lacking, as might health and exercise science students.

Individuals with both a health and exercise science background are not, however, the intended readers of the book. They are better served by reviewing specialized publications, such as those referenced in the book.

WHAT INFORMATION IS CONTAINED IN THE BOOK, HOW IS IT STRUCTURED, AND HOW MIGHT THE READER USE THE BOOK?

The book takes a lifespan approach. To describe how the different components of health might be altered by a given childhood-onset condition, the World Health Organization's International Classification of Functioning, Disability, and Health is used (World Health Organization 2001). According to the classification, *impairments* are problems with physiological functions (i.e. reduced control of voluntary movements) or anatomical parts (i.e. atypical brain, spinal cord, or muscle development), *activity limitations* are problems the individual might have in carrying out a task or an action (i.e. walking), and *participation restrictions* are problems involving situations encountered in real life (i.e. engaging in organized sporting events). *Functioning* is the individual's level of physiological and anatomical integrity, as well as their capacity to carry out activities and their participation performance, whereas *disability* is an umbrella term for the impairments, limitations, and restrictions. Since individuals exist within a particular context or contexts, based on their physical, social, and attitudinal environment, and their personal factors such as their sex, age, and experiences, how they may experience disability or how it might manifest for them can depend on their contextual factors in addition to their impairments, limitations, and restrictions (all of which can also influence each other). The book addresses common impairments and limitations that can restrict participation in physical activities as well as environmental barriers to physical activity participation and other issues related to their personal factors.

The book contains 12 chapters. The first five provide general information related to the promotion of physical fitness and activity, whereas the last eight present information specific to the various childhood-onset disabilities covered in the book. To avoid repetition, there is extensive referencing of the general chapters in the population-specific chapters. Tables, figures, and bullet points are used to facilitate quick access to information.

The following is an overview of the content and structure of the various chapters and how one might want to use the book.

Chapter 1 provides an overview of the book and how to use it and thus would be helpful to read first.

Chapter 2 can be considered an exercise science primer for people without such a background. It explains:

- The science underlying the health-related physical fitness components (cardiorespiratory endurance, muscular fitness, body composition, flexibility) that support engagement in physical activity (Caspersen et al. 1985);
- Why they are important;
- The principles of evaluating these components;
- The principles of training to improve them (cardiorespiratory endurance, muscular fitness) or the effect of physical activity on them (body composition, flexibility).

A review of the information in Chapter 2 will therefore help the reader understand the subsequent chapters and ultimately help the reader make informed decisions about fostering a lifestyle that promotes physical fitness and activity. The information in Chapter 2 is also referenced in the condition-specific chapters, which allows the reader to return to the fundamental information as required.

Chapter 3 discusses general safety issues that people with childhood-onset disabilities and their supporters should consider before the individual engages in cardiorespiratory endurance or muscular fitness evaluation or training, or in a more general physical activity programme or sport. This includes screening for readiness to engage in such activities, pain considerations, nutrition and hydration, common medications and their impact on physical activities, and precautions in the presence of common health issues that people with childhood-onset disability may face. The reader may wish to consider reviewing Chapter 3 after reviewing Chapter 2 or as needed when specific information in the chapter is referred to in the condition-specific chapters or when they are making physical fitness or activity-related decisions.

Chapter 4 discusses physical activity, as it relates to health in general and the different methods to measure it (i.e. directly watching what the person does, using questionnaires, having the person wear a small device that records their movement including their steps) as well as the strengths and limitations of these methods. The reader can use the information in Chapter 4 to work with physical activity professionals to determine the best tool for evaluating and tracking physical activity over time to help in designing and modifying a physical activity programme. The chapter could be read after Chapter 3 or when needed to help make decisions.

Chapter 5 explains the general principles for promoting a physically active lifestyle across the lifespan. Given physical activity is above all a behaviour, i.e. something the person does, the principles of promoting behavioural change and barriers and facilitators to physical activity behavioural change are described. Strategies are presented for overcoming barriers, including compensatory interventions such as the use of assistive devices and other technologies. The information in Chapter 5 can be used to help support motivation to increase physical activity, motivation being an important prerequisite for being physically active. The reader might read Chapter 5 after a review of Chapter 4 or before they are making decisions about a specific physical activity programme. The reader will also be referred back to Chapter 5 as relevant in each of the condition-specific chapters.

Chapters 6 to 12 each focus on one childhood-onset condition, a group, or related conditions. The conditions chosen for the book involve movement or developmental difficulties and there are therefore specific needs in terms of promoting physical fitness and activity. The conditions covered in the book, in order of appearance, are: cerebral palsy, developmental coordination disorder, spina bifida and childhood acquired spinal cord injury, childhood-onset neuromuscular conditions, intellectual disability, autism spectrum disorder, and juvenile idiopathic arthritis. To help in decision-making, each of these chapters contains, as relevant, condition-specific information on:

- The condition itself;
- Common medications and comorbidities (health issues) important to consider in the context of physical fitness and activity;
- The importance of physical fitness and activity;
- How physical fitness and activity might be measured;
- Principles of training to improve fitness and foster a physically active lifestyle.

In addition to this key information, some of the population-specific chapters also conclude with accounts from people living with a childhood-onset disability regarding their experiences of engaging in physical activities. The first-hand perspectives are meant to complement the information from experts. It is hoped the stories will inspire the reader's own creativity in finding solutions to any barriers to participation in physical activity, regardless of physical or other challenges.

REFERENCES

Caspersen CJ, Powell KE, Christenson GM (1985) Physical activity, exercise, and physical fitness: definitions and distinctions for health-related research. *Public Health Rep* **100**: 126–131.

World Health Organization (2001) *International Classification of Functioning, Disability and Health (ICF)*. Geneva, Switzerland: World Health Organization.

CHAPTER 2

Principles of Health-Related Physical Fitness Assessment and Training

Tim Takken, Olaf Verschuren, and Erik H Hulzebos

INTRODUCTION

Health professionals have acknowledged the importance and use of exercise in the prevention, diagnosis, and treatment of chronic medical conditions and related health problems (van Brussel et al. 2011). Health-related physical fitness is an important element of current and future health of individuals. Physical fitness is a multidimensional concept that has been defined as a set of attributes that people possess or achieve to perform physical activity (Caspersen et al. 1985). As opposed to persons without a disability, people with a chronic medical condition are often restricted in their participation in physical activities, including sports programmes, as a consequence of real or perceived impairments to body structures or processes, limitations to performing a physical task, and personal factors such as age, sex, level of education, and environmental barriers. The condition itself may often cause hypoactivity, which leads to a deconditioning effect, a reduction in functional ability, and further hypoactivity (Bar-Or and Rowland 2004). These individuals might end up in a vicious circle of decreasing physical fitness and functional abilities, leading to the additional risk of a variety of health conditions associated with a hypoactive lifestyle (e.g. obesity and diabetes).

In this chapter, we briefly review general methods for the evaluation of the different components of health-related fitness. Specific adaptations relevant to the various childhood-onset disabilities covered in this book can be found in the disability-specific chapters.

COMPONENTS OF HEALTH-RELATED PHYSICAL FITNESS

Physical fitness testing evaluates or measures health-related physical fitness. Health-related fitness relates to body structures (including the heart and lungs), muscle and movement, and the body's ability to release or store the energy obtained from food. Such energy is used to fuel body processes such as muscle contraction, which is essential for physical activity. The health-related components of physical fitness discussed in this chapter are cardiorespiratory fitness, muscular fitness, body composition, and flexibility.

Cardiorespiratory Fitness

When movement is longer than a few minutes, the energy from the food we eat is converted to a form of energy the body can use through chemical processes that require oxygen. Cardiorespiratory fitness is one measure of the body's capacity to perform physical activities that mainly depend on our oxygen-requiring energy system (e.g. walking, running, cycling, swimming, or propelling a wheelchair). With every breath we take, oxygen is taken up by the body and transported to tissues that need it. When we move, our active muscles and heart require additional energy and thus more oxygen than is needed at rest. Cardiorespiratory fitness is usually measured as the highest amount of oxygen that can be consumed by an individual during an exercise test during which the individual works at increasingly harder or more intense levels until exhaustion. The highest amount of oxygen consumption is called peak oxygen uptake. It is considered to be the single best indicator for cardiorespiratory fitness (Shephard et al. 1968). This one number is an indication of the integrated function of the lung, heart, and muscle (see Fig. 2.1). It is thus an important indicator of one's physical health.

Peak oxygen uptake depends somewhat on the test used to measure it. That means that a running test on a treadmill that requires the legs to work moving the whole body mass against gravity will lead to a peak oxygen uptake value that is 5% to 10% higher than a test for the same person that is performed on an exercise bicycle where the body mass is supported and most of the work is done by just the thigh muscles. In addition, arm muscles are smaller than leg muscles and use less oxygen. That means a test performed with the arms will give a lower peak oxygen uptake value (about 30%) compared to a test performed with the legs for the same person. So before comparing your 'number' with a friend's, it is important to know what test they did!

Most daily life activities do not require the highest amount of oxygen we can use. However, to understand how intense or hard a physical activity such as walking or running is, it is useful to compare one's peak oxygen uptake. Assume you and a friend of a similar

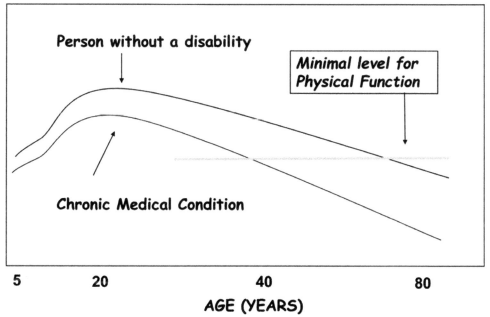

Figure 2.1 Model describing the development of cardiorespiratory fitness in individuals with and without disability

size and age are running at the same speed and are using the same amount of energy to run; however, you have a higher level of cardiorespiratory fitness (peak oxygen uptake). This means you will be using a lower proportion of your maximal capacity. Thus, the run will be relatively less intense for you compared to your friend. If the two of you have the same level of cardiorespiratory fitness, but you use less energy to run, you will again be using a lower proportion of your maximal capacity than your friend and the run will feel relatively less intense for you.

CARDIORESPIRATORY FITNESS TESTING IN CHILDREN VS ADULTS

Children's hearts, lungs, and circulatory responses to exercise are different from those of adults. This is largely because they are smaller than adults and thus have less muscle mass and smaller hearts and lungs. Two important responses that differ between adults and children are their heart rate, which is higher in children compared to adults, and peak oxygen uptake, which is lower in children than adults (Fig. 2.1). As can be seen in Figure 2.1, many chronic conditions have the same pattern of change in cardiorespiratory fitness with age. This increases as children age and thus grow, and decreases in adults as they grow older. People with a chronic condition start out with lower levels of fitness and the age-related decline is greater for them. This means the impact of age on their already compromised cardiorespiratory fitness is greater for individuals with a chronic condition than for someone without one.

MAXIMAL TESTS OF CARDIORESPIRATORY FITNESS

The criterion assessment to determine cardiorespiratory fitness (peak oxygen uptake) in an individual is by performing a test with an incremental work load (intensity) during exercise to exhaustion. During this test, the uptake of oxygen and output of carbon dioxide are measured using a respiratory gas analyser. Usually the individual breathes through a face mask or mouthpiece that is connected to the analyser. These tests are most often performed on a specialized exercise bicycle (cycle ergometer), a treadmill, or an arm-cranking device. There are many different protocols available to increase the workload during a test. The Bruce protocol on the treadmill and the Godfrey protocol on the cycle ergometer are among the most frequently used test protocols in children (Paridon et al. 2006). In adults the (modified) Bruce test for treadmill testing and the Wasserman RAMP protocol (Wasserman et al. 2005) for cycle ergometry are among the most frequently used test protocols.

There are several 'disability-specific' approaches to testing using a treadmill or a cycle ergometer. Examples of these are covered in the disability-specific chapters.

When one needs to test in the field, or when one does not have specialized equipment, one can estimate cardiorespiratory fitness using a 'field' test. The most frequently used field test globally is the shuttle run test. This test was developed by Leger et al. (1988) and can be used in both children and adults. In this test, an individual or group of people run back and forth in a gymnasium on a 20m track. The test starts with a running speed of 8km/hour and increases by 0.5km/hour every minute, with the speed guided by an external audio signal. An advantage of this test is that it can be performed in groups and that only simple equipment is required. A drawback is that the initial speed of 8km/hour might be too demanding for an individual with low cardiorespiratory fitness, including small children.

These tests, including field tests, usually last 6 to 10 minutes for children and 8 to 12 minutes for adolescents and adults. For the test to yield a meaningful value, it is important that the test reflect a maximum effort. To ensure the test is done to exhaustion, or that the individual is giving a maximal effort, the tester will provide verbal encouragement to the individual who is performing the test. In the population without any impairment, performing these tests to exhaustion is regarded as safe, including for children (Alpert et al. 1983) as long as proper safety precautions are taken into account and followed (Paridon et al. 2006). It is also important that the professional who conducts the test has sufficient competence and training to do so, and that the test selected is appropriate for the question being asked. That means that if one is interested in cardiorespiratory fitness related to running, one should use a treadmill test or a field test with running. For other safety information, we refer the reader to Chapter 3.

Submaximal Tests of Cardiorespiratory Fitness

Exercise tests that do not require the individual to exercise as hard as they are able (to exhaustion) have also been developed. These are called submaximal tests. They are used when a maximal test (one to exhaustion) is not the best option or feasible, typically in the general population because of a lack of equipment or expertise. Three submaximal tests often used are the Åstrand–Ryhming test (Åstrand and Ryhming 1954), the PWC170 test (Wahlund 1948), and the 6-minute walk test (ATS 2002).

The Åstrand-Ryhming test can be used to estimate peak oxygen uptake. During this test, the individual cycles for 6 minutes at a submaximal intensity with a heart rate of between 130 to 160 beats per minute on a cycle ergometer. Based on the person's sex, age, their work load (intensity), and the corresponding heart rate at the end of the 6-minute exercise, an estimate of peak oxygen uptake can be made using a mathematical formula derived from results from many people who have performed this test and a maximal test. Although the Åstrand-Ryhming test is widely used, the test result is highly influenced by the individual's resting heart rate. If you have a higher resting heart rate, your heart rate during exercise will also be higher. This means that the test would underestimate your peak oxygen uptake (cardiorespiratory fitness level). The reverse is also true, so this test is not necessarily appropriate for persons who use heart rate-lowering drugs (e.g. beta blockers) or who have an increased resting heart rate due a health issue or medication.

The PWC170 test was established more than 70 years ago by Wahlund (1948). The test is performed on a cycle ergometer up to a workload at which an exercise heart rate of 170 beat per minute is reached. The workload (intensity) at which the heart rate reaches 170 beats per minute is taken as an estimate for peak oxygen uptake. The PWC170 is established using different exercise protocols on a cycle ergometer. However, it is important to have a consistent heart rate during exercise, so the stages of the test should be at least 2 to 3 minutes in duration as the body needs this amount of time to have a consistent heart rate. These long duration stages can lead to a very long test in individuals who have high cardiorespiratory fitness. Given that there is a large difference in peak heart rate between individuals, possibly due to genetics or age (peak heart rate decreases as adults age), the heart rate of 170 beats per minute might be submaximal for one person but (near) maximal for another, meaning one cannot say that one of these people has a higher or lower cardiorespiratory fitness level than the other. As with the Åstrand-Ryhming test, increased or decreased resting heart rates can influence test results. So these two tests may be acceptable to track cardiorespiratory fitness in someone over the short-term but not over the long-term, and comparisons with others may be problematic.

The 6-minute walk test is a widely used submaximal field exercise test for measuring the ability to do a walking exercise. The individually typically walks back and forth on a 30m track in a hallway or gym. The test outcome is the distance walked in 6 minutes.

International guidelines exist regarding how to perform the test (Holland et al. 2014). Standard instructions and standard encouragements are also necessary as speed can change simply due to differences in instructions or encouragement. The test is often used with people with impairments (see Chapters 6 to 13) (de Groot and Takken 2011; Bartels et al. 2013). Unlike the other submaximal tests described above, the 6-minute walk test cannot be used to estimate peak oxygen uptake or cardiorespiratory fitness (Takken 2010), unless the person has a severely reduced walking capacity (i.e. less than 350m) (Lammers et al. 2011). Several sets of reference values have been established for both children (Mylius et al. 2016) and adults (Andrianopoulos et al. 2015). Walking distance is influenced by age, sex, weight, and height (leg length). In general, individuals without an impairment walk 500m to 700m in 6 minutes. It should also be noted that dividing the walk distance by 100 gives the individual's average walking speed (km/h) during the test. There is also a version of this test called the 6-minute ride test (Verschuren et al. 2013b) that can be performed using a wheelchair. More details can be obtained in Chapter 6.

TRAINING PRINCIPLES FOR CARDIORESPIRATORY FITNESS: CONSIDERATIONS

For the health care professional, it is important to have guidelines for selecting which individuals may benefit from an exercise training programme to improve cardiorespiratory fitness. We recommend using the so-called FITT factors (frequency, intensity, time, and type) as a guideline.

Training frequency refers to the number of exercise sessions per week. For children and adolescents with typical development, and for healthy adults, a training frequency of at least 3 to 5 sessions per week is recommended by the American College of Sports Medicine (ACSM) to increase and maintain cardiorespiratory fitness. It is a huge challenge to fit this into our busy lives (Garber et al. 2011). It should be noted that this is necessary to *improve* cardiorespiratory fitness. Fewer exercise or physical activity sessions per week may be sufficient if your goals are social or related to having a fun time (assuming you like exercise!) or if you simply want to be less inactive (sedentary).

Intensity refers to the effort of training (i.e. relative to your maximal capacity, meaning your level of cardiorespiratory fitness). Intensity is the most important factor for your training stimulus. The higher the intensity, the bigger and faster the training effect (change in cardiorespiratory fitness). With a higher intensity, you get bigger effects over the same (or even shorter) duration. However, these rapid improvements come with a down side: increased risk for discomfort, tiredness, and injuries. Exercise intensity is often prescribed relative to age-predicted maximal heart rate, heart rate reserve (the difference between a person's measured or predicted maximum heart rate and resting heart rate), and/or peak oxygen uptake as directly measured during a maximal graded exercise test. This intensity of training as recommended by the ACSM will give sufficient stimulus in many individuals (even those with an impairment) to improve their cardiorespiratory fitness (Garber et al. 2011). However, in individuals who are less fit for any reason, higher intensity may lead to more fatigue and slower recovery after an exercise session. Some individuals thus benefit from longer training programmes with a slower progression in intensity and session duration.

In terms of time, the current evidence from the ACSM guidelines (Garber et al. 2011) suggests that training sessions for aerobic fitness should be between 20 and 60 minutes. Although more may be better, at least 150 minutes of moderate to vigorous physical activities per week is advised. Training programmes should last for about 12 weeks consecutively. However, one can expect to see losses in cardiorespiratory fitness after training stops. So about 12 weeks after training, much of the gain may be gone. Most people who start exercising are not used to strenuous exercise, and they may need time to adapt to this higher level of activity. Therefore, we recommend a few weeks of training familiarization simply to reach the recommended training intensities. Longer interventions with progressive intensities (e.g. 12–16 weeks) may be useful. Importantly, greater doses of exercise are required to *improve* cardiorespiratory endurance than are needed to *maintain* these improvements.

With respect to type, to improve cardiorespiratory fitness, ACSM recommends regular purposeful exercise that involves major muscle groups and is continuous and rhythmic in nature (Garber et al. 2011). There are many types of activities, for example running, step-ups, taking stairs, fast walking, cycling, arm-cranking exercise, propelling a wheelchair, and swimming. Choose the activity that suits your needs, abilities, and preferences.

TRAINING FOR CARDIORESPIRATORY FITNESS: ADHERENCE

In our experience, adherence to exercise programmes may depend on individual motivation and thus in part on what activities are performed as well as on social support (i.e. we have found better adherence with exercise groups). We have also found that many individuals, including children and adolescents, often enjoy short-term, high-intensity exercises (when feasible) because they usually offer the necessary variation. Further, they better mimic the usual daily activity pattern, especially of children.

Adherence to an exercise programme might be very difficult for many previously inactive individuals to achieve but also to sustain the above exercise recommendations. It is very important to point out that it is very common for people to miss exercise sessions or even go through periods of complete attrition. Once a regular physical activity routine is established, however, short lapses in routine participation will have little or only modest influence on maintenance of cardiorespiratory fitness (Garber et al. 2011).

Muscular Fitness: Overview

Muscular fitness is the ability of the muscle to generate strength for a certain period of time. It consists of muscular strength (maximal force that muscle can produce) and muscular endurance, namely the capacity of the muscle to contract for a given time at a non-maximal or submaximal level (American College of Sports Medicine 2013).

In general, there are three types of muscle contractions: isometric, concentric, and eccentric muscle strength:

1. Isometric contractions: an individual generates a muscle contraction; however, because external resistance is higher, there is no shortening of the muscle. This is the case when you are pushing against a wall.
2. Concentric contractions: an individual generates a muscle contraction that results in shortening of the muscle. This is the case when you are lifting a load.
3. Eccentric contractions: an individual generates a muscle contraction; however, the muscle lengthens under an external load. This is the case in the muscles that straighten your knees when you are walking down the stairs.

Muscle Fitness: Muscle Strength

Because of these differences in muscular contractions, different muscle strength tests on the same muscle group will provide a different result – hence, it is important to be clear what question is driving the testing. In general, isometric muscle strength tests provide the highest value for a muscle group. For eccentric muscle strength, the number of repetitions is important. The load or weight that a muscle group can 'lift' only one time in a row (before fatigue) is called the one-repetition maximum for the muscle group in question. This is considered the standard way to measure muscle strength.

Muscle strength is often considered as 'the glue that holds us together'. For many activities in daily life, a certain threshold of muscle strength is required. If you have strength above this threshold you do not perceive limitations in performing the activity, and more strength does not result in better function of the task. However, once you fall below this threshold, muscle strength may become a factor that limits your ability to perform the task. Muscle mass is an important factor for muscle strength. The more muscle mass you have, the stronger you are in general. However, an important factor that is often overlooked is coordination. Coordination of a muscle group is very important for efficient movement. In the first weeks of training almost all improvements in muscle strength are due to improved muscle coordination as opposed to muscles growing larger (hypertrophy) (Garber et al. 2011).

TESTS OF MUSCLE STRENGTH

Two methods to assess isometric muscle strength are manual muscle testing and use of a hand-held dynamometry. *Manual muscle testing* uses an ordinal 6-point (0–5) scale such as the Medical Research Council scale (Medical Research Council 1981). This type of testing is usually most accurate when muscles are weak. *Hand-held dynamometry* consists of a simple hand-held device equipped with a small internal load cell capable of measuring muscular force (e.g. newton). Isokinetic dynamometry, most often used in a research or advanced clinical setting, uses computer-controlled equipment to measure the muscular force generated throughout a controlled movement. Isokinetic assessment has several advantages over isometric testing. Most activities of daily living involve phases of dynamic muscle action, and in this sense isokinetic testing may provide more specificity in terms of muscle action type than isometric testing. On the other hand, a maximal isometric contraction is only indicative of the capacity to produce force in that condition and at that particular muscle length, and cannot necessarily be extrapolated to conditions where the muscle length is different or changing throughout the task. Perhaps most important, however, is the inherent safety of isokinetic actions, afforded by the computer-controlled mechanism of accommodating resistance against which the muscle contracts.

So, there is a wide range of procedures available. Sometimes tests have to be modified for children given their size and ability to follow instructions. Details for using a hand-held dynamometer or an isokinetic device for children as well as how well these tests can determine change can be found elsewhere (Wright et al. 2012). Reference values for isometric muscle strength of the arm and leg muscles for children and adolescents, measured using a hand-held dynamometer, are also available (Hebert et al. 2015). Adult procedures and reference data have also at times been used with children (Jones and Stratton 2000). More functionally based strength tests can also be performed. One example is the 'repetition maximum test'. The individual can repeatedly stand from a squat with additional weights to measure strength of the muscles that straighten the legs, for example. With this test, the number of repetitions to fatigue (not being able to continue) is noted. For example, the weight at which an individual can perform 15 repetitions to fatigue is called the 15-repetition maximum. This test can be used for evaluation (meaning the number of repetitions is predetermined), and the weight at that number of repetitions is found. The weight can also be translated back to a percentage of the person's one repetition maximum.

All of the above tests required skilled evaluators to ensure that the values obtained reflect the person's real muscle strength. With manual muscles testing and hand-held dynamometry, the tests can also be limited by the maximal strength of the tester. This means the test may not be feasible for particularly strong individuals. To overcome this problem with hand-held dynamometry, straps can be used (Hebert et al. 2011).

When skilled evaluators or specialized equipment are not available, age-appropriate standardized motor tasks (functional activities like the broad jump or standing long jump) can be used to estimate the strength of groups of muscles working together to perform the task.

TRAINING PRINCIPLES FOR MUSCLE STRENGTH: CONSIDERATIONS

Strength training procedures are different for children and adults. In adults, one of the most effective ways to increase muscle strength is by a low number of repetitions and a high weight (4–6 repetitions to exhaustion). However, in young people the biggest improvement is found when they do more repetitions with a lower weight (8–12 repetitions) to exhaustion (Lloyd et al. 2014) (see Table 2.1).

In children who have not reached puberty, the largest gain in muscle strength with training is due to an improvement in neuromuscular coordination of the muscle contractions, meaning, essentially, they become stronger because they become more skilled at contracting their muscles, rather than because their muscles have become larger. Because children before puberty have low levels of hormones like testosterone that support muscle growth, they do not show a great deal of increase in muscle mass with strength training. With individuals who are not familiar with strength training, it is important first to focus on proper technique, so they develop the motor skills necessary to train safely. Only after proper technique is developed should the focus be shifted to lifting more weight. This focus on technique and skills will also reduce the risk for musculoskeletal injuries.

The following describes the muscle strength training considerations of frequency, intensity, volume, time or duration and the type of exercise.

For children and healthy adults, recommendations call for a training frequency of two to three times per week on non-consecutive days. This allows for sufficient recuperation between the sessions. More than four times per week does not give additional gain in strength, at least not in children (Lloyd et al. 2014).

In terms of training intensity, according to the ACSM guidelines (Garber et al. 2011), novice individuals should use a load (weight) that allows no more than 10 to 15

Table 2.1 Training parameters for increasing muscle strength in children and adolescents

Parameter	
Frequency	2–3/wk
Intensity	≤80% of 1 repetition maximum
Time	30–60min per session for at least 8–20wks
Type	Single-joint machine-based exercises to machine plus free-weight, multi-joint resistance exercises
Repetitions	6–12
Sets	2–4
Number of different exercises	6–8

Source: Adapted from main body of text in Lloyd et al. (2014).

repetitions before fatigue (i.e. 60%–75% of the one repetition maximum load or weight) for one to two sets to be completed, without undue muscle fatigue. For adults without a disability 8 to 12 repetitions are recommended.

Volume of training refers to the total number of work sets performed per session (i.e. not including warm-up sets). According to the ACSM guidelines for novice exercisers (Garber et al. 2011), the load should be sufficient to allow no more than 6 to 15 repetitions before muscle fatigue and performed for one to three sets. More than two sets are recommended if you want to increase the endurance of your muscles as opposed to the muscle strength (Faigenbaum and Myer 2010), in which case intensity rather than volume should be the focus (Garber et al. 2011).

As for time or duration, guidelines (Garber et al. 2011) state that a short-term resistance programme for young people should last at least 8 to 20 weeks. This is recommended because people new to strength training are not used to strenuous exercise and may need time to adapt to this level of activity. Therefore, we recommend a few weeks of strength training familiarization simply to reach the recommended training volumes and intensities. Longer interventions with progressive intensities (e.g. 12–16 weeks) may be needed to experience significant or meaningful improvements in muscle strength. Once training is stopped, however, strength may decrease, so a maintenance programme may be useful.

In terms of the type of exercise, single-joint strength training may be more effective for very weak individuals or for children, adolescents, and adults who are new to strength training, particularly at the initial phases of training. This type of exercise may also be best for adults who tend to compensate when performing multi-joint exercises using both arms or legs at once. Individuals who are not able to walk independently might also benefit from strength training, but they may lack the selective motor control needed to perform single-joint exercises. Functionally based strength training, similar to functionally based strength testing, may be the most feasible for them.

Muscular Fitness: Muscular Endurance (*Anaerobic Fitness*)

The ability to perform short duration (<30s) physical exercise is called anaerobic fitness and is a type of muscular endurance. Anaerobic means without oxygen. In other words, the energy system that the body uses for this type of activity does not require oxygen. The shorter the exercise lasts, the higher the intensity of the exercise can be. So, for example, if the distance is shorter, you can run at a higher speed than if the distance is longer.

Anaerobic fitness is assumed to be an especially relevant health-related fitness outcome in children because most activities of daily living of children are characterized by intermittent short bursts of intensive exercise. Anaerobic fitness is also important for many types of sports, like team sports such as football, basketball, and ice hockey. In these sports, short bursts (15–30s) of high-intensity activity are intertwined with periods of low intensity (active rest).

Tests of Anaerobic Fitness

WINGATE ANAEROBIC TESTS (CYCLE AND ARM-CRANK VERSIONS)

In the laboratory setting, anaerobic fitness is usually measured using the Wingate Anaerobic test. This is a 30-second all-out test on an exercise bicycle (cycle ergometer) (Bar-Or 1987) or on an arm-crank device (arm ergometer) for the Wingate arm-cranking test (Verschuren et al. 2013c). Because of the high intensity of these tests, the energy sources in your working muscles are used at a fast rate, and fatigue occurs within a few seconds. Because of this, the 30-second test is perceived as being quite long for the person performing it. The test has been considered as challenging, but generally feasible if one has the motor skills to perform it. One of the drawbacks of these tests is that a special cycle or arm ergometer is required as well as special software to measure the power output (the intensity or how hard the person is working over time). Different devices might also use different methods to obtain the actual highest power output (called peak power) and the average power during the 30 seconds (called the mean power, which is also considered an evaluation for muscle endurance). From a practical standpoint, rather than use reference values, it may be more helpful to track individual progress over time if this test is to be used.

In addition to costly equipment and specialized software, the Wingate Anaerobic tests also require specialized training for the tester. Because of these drawbacks, field tests for anaerobic fitness are often used. Two examples for lower limb muscles for children are the Muscle Power Sprint Test (6 × 15m sprint), and the 10 × 5m sprint test (Verschuren et al. 2007, 2013a). Reference values are available for typically developing children for the Muscle Power Sprint Test (Steenman et al. 2016). Examples for the lower limb muscles for adults are the Running-Based Anaerobic Sprint Test (6 × 35m) and also the 10 × 5m sprint can be used (Draper and Whyte 1997; Verschuren et al. 2007).

TRAINING PRINCIPLES FOR ANAEROBIC FITNESS: CONSIDERATIONS

A new exercise training paradigm in clinical exercise physiology is high-intensity interval training (HIIT). Although interval training has been used by athletes for many decades, it has only recently attracted attention to clinical populations. During HIIT, there is a systematic alternation between work (exercise) and (active) recovery. This alternation gives an effective training stimulus to skeletal muscles and the heart.

Many studies on people without a disability, as well as clinical populations, have shown that HIIT is an effective training paradigm that produces a large effect in quite a short time frame (Gibala 2007; Wisloff et al. 2009; Bacon et al. 2013). In principle, an unlimited number of combinations between duration and intensity of intervals and active rest

Table 2.2 Training parameters for anaerobic high-intensity interval training in children and adolescents

Parameter	
Frequency	2–4/wk
Intensity	90–100% of maximal intensity/running speed (sprint)
Repetitions	5–10
Time	Work: 20–30s
	Active rest: 60–90s
Series	4–5
Duration of programme	8–13wks

Recommendations are based on Baquet et al. (2003) and Klijn et al. (2003).

can be made. However, it has been suggested that longer intervals might be less effective in children. Therefore, for children and adolescents short and intensive sprints of approximately 30 seconds are recommended (anaerobic HIIT; see Table 2.2 for details). For adults this approach is also effective; however, intervals with a longer duration and lower intensity are recommended, making it more of an aerobic (cardiorespiratory fitness) HIIT. In this training approach intervals have a duration of about 4 minutes (see Table 2.3 for details).

Body Composition

Body composition is another component of physical fitness. How much of your weight is muscle tissue, how much is fat tissue, and how much is bone? Body composition is important for your performance in physical activities and current health but also

Table 2.3 Training parameters for aerobic high-intensity interval training in adults

Parameter	
Frequency	3/wk
Intensity	Work: 90–95% of maximal heart rate
	Recovery: 50–70% of maximal heart rate
Repetitions	4
Time	Work: 4min
	Recovery: 3min
Series	1
Type	Walking, cycling
Duration of programme	12wks

Source: Adapted from main body of text in Wisloff et al. (2009).

for healthy ageing. Too much fat tissue is unhealthy for your heart and blood vessels. Individuals who are overweight or obese have too high a fat mass and have a greater risk of dying prematurely (Calle et al. 2005). Also, having too high a fat mass can make it harder to perform physical activity as it takes more energy to move a heavier person than a lighter person (especially when activates are against gravity or are not weight-supported, such as walking or running). Muscle mass is also an important factor for performing physical activities because strength is dependent on the amount of muscle mass. Also, one's cardiorespiratory endurance is related to muscle mass. The more muscle mass you have, the more mitochondria you have (small energy plants in your muscles that convert nutrients into energy). These mitochondria make energy for your muscle contractions. Thus, the more you have (and the better they work), the more muscle contractions you can make, and the faster you can exercise! The reference values for percentage of fat mass for young male adults are 13% to 20% and for older male adults are 22.5% to 29.3% (Coin et al. 2008). For young female adults reference values are 26.1% to 35%, and for older female adults they are 32.5% to 40% (Coin et al. 2008).

Bone mass is also important. While one gains bone mass during childhood (especially during puberty), one only loses bone mass after puberty. Weight-bearing exercise can slow down this loss. Therefore, weight-bearing exercise such as walking and running is important for bone health.

Tests of Body Composition

When accuracy is very important, specialized tests are done. The criterion standards for body composition are reference methods such as isotope dilution, dual-energy X-ray absorptiometry, magnetic resonance imaging, or hydrostatic weighing. These methods require sophisticated and expensive equipment. Of these, dual-energy X-ray absorptiometry scans are the most accurate and accessible measure of body composition and considered the criterion standard. These are typically conducted within the hospital setting to measure bone mass but also report on muscle and fat mass. Dual-energy X-ray absorptiometry scans require trained technicians and provide a small dose of radiation – so should not be conducted frequently.

Skinfold measurement and bioelectrical impedance analysis are techniques to estimate body composition (Durnin and Rahaman 1967; Jackson et al. 1988). There are several sites to measure skinfolds. The tester must closely follow the exact instructions of the method being used to obtain an accurate result. Typically, four sites are measured: these are on the front and back of the upper back and at the hip. Because skinfold measurements are site-specific, there might be some difference between testers if the sites are not exactly the same. Experience with the technique is important to obtain accurate results. Skinfold measurement and its conversion to percentage of body fat may also be imprecise in some persons, especially those at the extremes of the normal distribution (e.g. those individuals with high or low percentages of body fat). The measurement of bioimpedance (which measures total body water by passing a small electrical current through the body, and then uses total body water to estimate calculate body composition) is less influenced by the tester than the measure of skinfolds. However, changes in the bioimpedance outcome might be influenced by hydration status, prior exercise, etc. Anything that changes your body fluid volume interferes with the test result. Standardization (e.g. same time of day, tested in fasted state, no strenuous exercise) is important to be able to compare results.

A common body composition measure that requires little equipment is body mass index (BMI), which is your weight divided by your height squared (height × height) Although used for the assessment of overweight (BMI between 25 and 30 for adults) or obesity (BMI >30 for adults), BMI has some limitations. A high BMI can be found in individuals with a high muscle mass or high levels of body fat. In addition, for children, there is not one value that determines whether one is likely to be overweight or obese. The relevant values change with sex and age, and are usually shown as centiles for a given age and sex. Overweight is considered to be the 85th to less than the 95th centile, and obese is considered to be equal to or greater than the 95th centile (Centers for Disease Control and Prevention 2017b). The American Centers for Disease Control and Prevention has an online programme that allows one to calculate one's centile (referred to as a percentile) score for one's age and sex (Centers for Disease Control and Prevention 2017a).

Effects of Physical Activity on Body Composition

Although often stated, the effect of physical activity on the body's level of fat (fat mass) is limited. Fat is a very energy-dense tissue. This means that you have to expend a lot of energy (long and intense workouts) before you can lose 1kg of fat. The good news is that although body mass does not change with a large increase in physical activity, body composition can improve. You get a higher muscle mass and a somewhat lower fat mass with exercise. While this might not change your BMI, your fat percentage is lower and your muscle percentage is higher meaning an overall healthier body composition.

Flexibility

Flexibility refers to the range of motion of a body part. Flexibility is an important factor for daily function. A limited range of motion will reduce the ability to perform certain activities. Although it is often stated that flexibility is important for injury prevention, research shows that doing flexibility exercises does not reduce the risk for the occurrence of activity-related injuries (Garber et al. 2011).

Tests of Flexibility

Flexibility is often tested using the measurement of active or passive range of motion. Active range of motion refers to the range of movement of an individual during voluntary activities. Passive range of motion refers to the range of movement during an activity when someone else provides external power to measure the range of motion. Passive range of motion is often larger than the active range of motion.

Precise flexibility measures can be taken using a double-armed electronic goniometer. This goniometer provides the range of motion of a certain joint. Physiotherapists often measure flexibility using a manual goniometer. Similarly, an inclinometer can be used to measure joint angles. Functional or field tests can also be used, of which one example is the sit and reach test. This tests the flexibility of your back and hamstring muscles (muscles on the back of the thigh). Examples of reference values for the sit and reach test are 24.3cm ± 13.2cm for female adults and 18.9cm ± 12.0cm for male adults (Garber et al. 2011).

EFFECTS OF PHYSICAL ACTIVITY ON FLEXIBILITY

ACSM recommends performing flexibility exercises at least 2 to 3 days per week (Garber et al. 2011), with the greatest gains achieved when the exercises are performed daily. Stretch your muscle to the point of tightness or slight discomfort and hold this for 10 to 30 seconds. It is recommended to stretch all major muscle groups. The best effects are obtained when the muscle is sufficiently pre-warmed using light aerobic exercise (e.g. walking, running in place) or a warm bath or shower.

CONCLUSION

Health-related physical fitness components such as cardiorespiratory fitness, muscular fitness body composition, and flexibility are important indicators for your current and future health. In this chapter, we have provided advice regarding approaches to measurement as well as methods to improve these fitness components in the general population. For disability-specific information, the reader is referred to the specific chapters for each disability covered in this book.

REFERENCES

Alpert BS, Verrill DE, Flood NL, Boineau JP, Strong WB (1983) Complications of ergometer exercise in children. *Pediatr Cardiol* 4: 91–96.

American College of Sports Medicine (2013) *ACSM's Health-Related Physical Fitness Assessment Manual.* Baltimore: Lippincott Williams & Wilkins.

Andrianopoulos V, Holland AE, Singh SJ et al. (2015) Six-minute walk distance in patients with chronic obstructive pulmonary disease: which reference equations should we use? *Chron Respir Dis* 12: 111–119. 10.1177/1479972315575201.

Åstrand P-O, Ryhming I (1954) A nomogram for calculation of aerobic capacity (physical fitness) from pulse rate during submaximal work. *Journal of Applied Physiology* 7: 218–221.

ATS (2002) ATS statement: guidelines for the six-minute walk test. *Am J Respir Crit Care Med* **166**: 111–117.

Bacon AP, Carter RE, Ogle EA, Joyner MJ (2013) VO2max trainability and high intensity interval training in humans: a meta-analysis. *PLoS One* **8**: e73182. 10.1371/journal.pone.0073182.

Baquet G, Van Praagh E, Berthoin S (2003) Endurance training and aerobic fitness in young people. *Sports Med* **33**: 1127–1143.

Bar-Or O (1987) The Wingate anaerobic test: an update on methodology, reliability and validity. *Sports Med* **4**: 381–394.

Bar-Or O, Rowland TW (2004) *Pediatric Exercise Medicine: From Physiologic Principles to Healthcare Application.* Champaign: Human Kinetics.

Bartels B, De Groot JF, Terwee CB (2013) The six-minute walk test in chronic pediatric conditions: a systematic review of measurement properties. *Phys Ther* **93**: 529–541. 10.2522/ptj.20120210.

Calle EE, Teras LR, Thun MJ (2005) Obesity and mortality. *New England Journal of Medicine* **353**: 2197–2199. 10.1056/nejm200511173532020.

Caspersen CJ, Powel KE, Christenson GM (1985) Physical activity, exercise, and physical fitness: definitions and distinctions for health-related research. *Public Health Rep* **100**: 126–131.

Centers for Disease Control and Prevention (2017a) *BMI Percentile Calculator for Child and Teen English Version* [online]. Available at: https://www.cdc.gov/healthyweight/bmi/calculator.html [Accessed 23 November 2017].

Centers for Disease Control and Prevention (2017b) *Child and Teen BMI* [online]. Available at: https://www.cdc.gov/healthyweight/assessing/bmi/childrens_bmi/about_childrens_bmi.html [Accessed November 23 2017].

Coin A, Sergi G, Minicuci N et al. (2008) Fat-free mass and fat mass reference values by dual-energy X-ray absorptiometry (DEXA) in a 20–80-year-old Italian population. *Clin Nutr* **27**: 87–94. 10.1016/j.clnu.2007.10.008.

De Groot JF, Takken T (2011) The six-minute walk test in paediatric populations. *J Physiother* **57**: 128. 10.1016/S1836-9553(11)70026-1.

Draper N, Whyte G (1997) Here's a new running based test of anaerobic performance for which you need only a stopwatch and a calculator. *Peak Performance* **96**: 3–5.

Durnin JV, Rahaman MM (1967) The assessment of the amount of fat in the human body from measurements of skinfold thickness. *Br J Nutr* **21**: 681–689.

Faigenbaum AD, Myer GD (2010) Pediatric resistance training: benefits, concerns, and program design considerations. *Curr Sports Med Rep* **9**: 161–168. 10.1249/JSR.0b013e3181de1214.

Garber CE, Blissmer B, Deschenes MR et al. (2011) American College of Sports Medicine position stand: quantity and quality of exercise for developing and maintaining cardiorespiratory, musculoskeletal, and neuromotor fitness in apparently healthy adults: guidance for prescribing exercise. *Med Sci Sports Exerc* **43**: 1334–1359. 10.1249/MSS.0b013e318213fefb.

Gibala MJ (2007) High-intensity interval training: a time-efficient strategy for health promotion? *Curr Sports Med Rep* **6**: 211–213.

Hebert LJ, Maltais DB, Lepage C, Saulnier J, Crete M (2015) Hand-held dynamometry isometric torque reference values for children and adolescents. *Pediatr Phys Ther* **27**: 414–423. 10.1097/PEP.0000000000000179.

Hebert LJ, Maltais DB, Lepage C, Saulnier J, Crete M, Perron M (2011) Isometric muscle strength in youth assessed by hand-held dynamometry: a feasibility, reliability, and validity study. *Pediatr Phys Ther* **23**: 289–299. 10.1097/PEP.0b013e318227ccff.

Holland AE, Spruit MA, Troosters T et al. (2014) An official European Respiratory Society/American Thoracic Society technical standard: field walking tests in chronic respiratory disease. *Eur Respir J* **44**: 1428–1446. 10.1183/09031936.00150314.

Jackson AS, Pollock ML, Graves JE, Mahar MT (1988) Reliability and validity of bioelectrical impedance in determining body composition. *J Appl Physiol* **64**: 529–534.

Jones M, Stratton G (2000) Muscle function assessment in children. *Acta Paediatrica* **89**: 753–761.

Klijn PH, Terheggen-Lagro SW, Van der Ent CK, Van der Net J, Kimpen JL, Helders PJ (2003) Anaerobic exercise in pediatric cystic fibrosis. *Pediatric Pulmonology* **36**: 223–229.

Lammers AE, Diller GP, Odendaal D, Tailor S, Derrick G, Haworth SG (2011) Comparison of 6-min walk test distance and cardiopulmonary exercise test performnce in children with pulmonary hypertension. *Arch Dis Child* **96**: 141–147.

Leger LA, Mercier D, Gadoury C, Lambert J (1988) The multistage 20 metre shuttle run test for aerobic fitness. *J Sports Sci* **6**: 93–101.

Lloyd RS, Faigenbaum AD, Stone MH et al. (2014) Position statement on youth resistance training: the 2014 International Consensus. *Br J Sports Med* **48**: 498–505. 10.1136/bjsports-2013-092952.

Medical Research Council (1981) *Aids to the Examination of the Peripheral Nervous System, Memorandum No. 45.* London: Her Majesty's Stationery Office.

Mylius CF, Paap D, Takken T (2016) Reference value for the 6-minute walk test in children and adolescents: a systematic review. *Expert Rev Respir Med* **10**: 1335–1352. 10.1080/17476348.2016.1258305.

Paridon SM, Alpert BS, Boas SR et al. (2006) Clinical stress testing in the pediatric age group: a statement from the American Heart Association Council on Cardiovascular Disease in the Young, Committee on Atherosclerosis, Hypertension, and Obesity in Youth. *Circulation* **113**: 1905–1920.

Shephard RJ, Allen C, Benade AJ et al. (1968) The maximum oxygen intake. An international reference standard of cardiorespiratory fitness. *Bull World Health Organ* **38**: 757–764.

Steenman K, Verschuren O, Rameckers E, Douma-Van Riet D, Takken T (2016) Extended reference values for the muscle power sprint test in 6- to 18-year-old children. *Pediatr Phys Ther* **28**: 78–84. 10.1097/PEP.0000000000000209.

Takken T (2010) Six-minute walk test is a poor predictor of maximum oxygen uptake in children. *Acta Paediatr* **99**: 958; author reply 958–959. 10.1111/j.1651-2227.2010.01750.x.

Van Brussel M, Van der Net J, Hulzebos E, Helders PJ, Takken T (2011) The Utrecht approach to exercise in chronic childhood conditions: the decade in review. *Pediatr Phys Ther* **23**: 2–14. 10.1097/PEP.0b013e318208cb22.

Verschuren O, Bongers BC, Obeid J, Ruyten T, Takken T (2013a) Validity of the muscle power sprint test in ambulatory youth with cerebral palsy. *Pediatr Phys Ther* **25**: 25–28. 10.1097/PEP.0b013e3182791459.

Verschuren O, Ketelaar M, De Groot J, Vila Nova F, Takken T (2013b) Reproducibility of two functional field exercise tests for children with cerebral palsy who self-propel a manual wheelchair. *Dev Med Child Neurol* **55**: 185–190. 10.1111/dmcn.12052.

Verschuren O, Takken T, Ketelaar M, Gorter J, Helders, P (2007) Reliability for running tests for measuring agility and anaerobic muscle power in children and adolescents with cerebral palsy. *Pediatr Phys Ther* **19**: 108–115. 00001577-200701920-00002 [pii].

Verschuren O, Zwinkels M, Obeid J, Kerkhof N, Ketelaar M, Takken T (2013c) Reliability and validity of short-term performance tests for wheelchair-using children and adolescents with cerebral palsy. *Dev Med Child Neurol* **55**: 1129–1135. 10.1111/dmcn.12214.

Wahlund H (1948) Determination of the physical working capacity. *Acta Medica Scandinavica* **215**: 1–78.

Wasserman K, Hansen JE, Sue DY, Casaburi R, Whipp BJ (2005) *Principles of Exercise Testing and Interpretation.* Baltimore, MD: Lippincott, Williams & Wilkins.

Wisloff U, Ellingsen O, Kemi OJ (2009) High-intensity interval training to maximize cardiac benefits of exercise training? *Exercise and Sport Science Reviews* **37**: 139–146. 10.1097/JES.0b013e3181aa65fc.

Wright FW, Maltais DB, Sanders H, Burtner PA (2012) Neuromusculoskeletal and movement-related functions. In: Majnemer A, editor, *Measures for Children with Developmental Disabilities: An ICF-CY Approach.* London: Mac Keith Press, pp 192–230.

CHAPTER 3

Safety Considerations

Haakon Dalen and Reidun B Jahnsen

SCREENING FOR CONTRAINDICATIONS TO PHYSICAL ACTIVITY

Physical activity is not only beneficial, but of vital importance for well-being and overall health for all children and adults; it is of special importance for children with a chronic health condition. The same applies for adults with a lifelong history of a chronic health condition. Importantly, chronic health conditions can affect both cognitive and physical function, and adjustments and modifications of the activities and exercises may be needed (Bauman et al. 2002; Garber et al. 2011; Kohl et al. 2012; American College of Sports Medicine et al. 2016).

There are few if any strict general contraindications to physical activity in persons with chronic health conditions, and the adjustments and modifications are mostly related to special conditions or medical concerns, for instance heart disease (Franklin and Billecke 2012; Fletcher et al. 2013; American College of Sports Medicine et al. 2016). The screening usually takes place in ordinary medical consultations, based on a longitudinal relationship between the doctor, child, and the family, and provides the doctor with both the health history of the person and their current health status (Goodman et al. 2011; American College of Sports Medicine et al. 2014; Riebe et al. 2015). Regarding children, there is no single medical assessment or health record that encompasses an overview of all of a child's medical and developmental needs, and a medical assessment should always include a comprehensive history of the child's medical, social, and developmental needs. Most children with childhood-onset disabilities present an extensive medical history of tests and examinations, and there would seldom be any need for additional laboratory testing and examination (Myer et al. 2011; American College of Sports Medicine et al. 2016). There are several types of consultative examinations, that is psychiatric, mental status, orthopaedic/musculoskeletal, internal medicine, neurological, and other specialized evaluations (Goodman et al. 2011; American College of Sports Medicine et al. 2014; Riebe et al. 2015).

It is important to take into account differences in personality and achievement between individuals. It is vital to emphasize the strengths of the individual and their family, not simply the problems and procedures. Assessments should address the holistic needs of the individual and the family, and the focus should always be on what they *can do*, and not what they *cannot do* (Goodman et al. 2011; American College of Sports Medicine et al. 2014; Riebe et al. 2015; American College of Sports Medicine et al. 2016).

In recommending physical activities, some may need to be avoided because of the increased risk of injury specific to the condition (American College of Sports Medicine et al. 2016).

PAIN

Pain is a subjective experience, and only the person who experiences pain can express or describe it. The International Association for the Study of Pain (IASP) defines chronic pain as 'an unpleasant sensory and emotional experience associated with actual or potential tissue damage, or described in terms of such damage' (Merskey and Bogduk 1994).

Assessing pain in persons with disabilities or impairments, whether developmental, cognitive, or physical, presents special challenges, particularly in children (Merkel et al. 1997; Hadden and von Baeyer 2002). It may also be a challenge to understand the experience of adults with intellectual disability or communication difficulties. Self-assessment is always recommended, but depending on the severity and type of disability this may not be possible in some cases. Instead one may need to rely on caregiver reports, physiological measures, and/or observed behaviour of the person. Some of the behaviours that indicate pain in a child include whether the child is cranky, seeking comfort, and gesturing to a part of the body that hurts. One should watch for decreased physical activity, changes in sleep pattern or appetite, irritability, crankiness, unruly behaviour, or non-verbal expressions of pain, such as wincing, gasping, or frowning (Merkel et al. 1997; Hadden and von Baeyer 2002).

There are several instruments assessing pain, and faces scales have become the most popular for eliciting children's self-reports of pain. In a systematic review, 14 faces pain scales were identified, of which four have undergone extensive psychometric testing: Faces Pain Scale (scored 0–6); Faces Pain Scale-Revised (0–10); Oucher pain scale (0–10); and Wong–Baker Faces Pain Rating Scale (0–10) (Tomlinson et al. 2010). The authors conclude that there is no need to change to another pain scale if any of those four scales are in use, but the children prefer the Wong–Baker Scale (Tomlinson et al. 2010). However, the children rate higher pain intensity when the non-pain face is smiling, which is a disadvantage of this scale. The Faces Pain Scale-Revised is recommended for research purposes (Tomlinson et al. 2010).

One commonly used strategy for assessing pain in children is QUESTT: **Q**uestion the child; **U**se a pain rating scale; **E**valuate the behaviour and physiological changes; **S**ecure parents' involvement; **T**ake cause of pain into account; **T**ake action and evaluate results (Wong and Baker 1988).

In adults with a lifelong history of disability, pain is one of the most common symptoms and problems (Jahnsen et al. 2004). In a state of persistent pain, adults may limit what they do, either because activity exacerbates the pain or because they are afraid of re-injury or falling. However, in the case of persistent pain that limits activity, a vicious circle of restriction, decreased participation, and greater disability may result, and may also lead to chronic problems in initiating and maintaining sleep. In cerebral palsy (CP), which is the most common cause of motor impairments in children, musculo-skeletal pain is a dominant problem, both in children and adults (Jahnsen et al. 2004; Ramstad et al. 2011) (see Chapter 6). For children with CP it may partly be due to the inherent deficits associated with the condition, as well as with the invasive medical and surgical procedures and rehabilitative activities they undergo on a regular basis (Ramstad et al. 2011). For adults, pain is associated with both overuse and inactivity (Jahnsen et al. 2004).

Pain that arises from actual or threatened damage to non-neural tissues is due to the activation of nociceptors. This term is designed to contrast with neuropathic pain. It is used to describe pain occurring with a typically functioning somatosensory nervous system, to contrast with the atypical function seen in neuropathic pain (Russo et al. 2008).

Neuropathic pain can be divided into central and peripheral neuropathic pain, dependent on whether the origin of the lesion or disease is in the central or the peripheral nervous system (IASP 2004). Neuropathic pain is a common problem in both children and adults with childhood-onset disabilities. It is a complex, chronic pain state that is usually accompanied by tissue injury. With neuropathic pain, the nerve fibres themselves might be damaged, dysfunctional, or injured (IASP 2004). It is very hard to treat effectively, but physical activity very seldom represents any contraindication. On the contrary, purposeful activities can be an effective tool in focusing the attention on things other than pain. In addition, several experimental studies indicate that exercise helps to alleviate neuropathic pain by reducing levels of certain inflammation-promoting factors (IASP 2004).

NUTRITION AND HYDRATION CONSIDERATIONS

Many children with childhood-onset disabilities are at risk of poor nutritional status, particularly those with significant gross motor impairment and oropharyngeal dysfunction. It may result in reduced skeletal development, including decreased linear growth and bone mineral density compared to typically developing people (Sullivan et al.

2000). Nutritional requirements must be established, but estimating the nutritional needs for an individual with neurological impairment is not straightforward. Accurate estimations are difficult because of variations in energy requirements related to the heterogeneity of the group, altered body composition, and reduced physical activity levels. However, persons with different physical and/or intellectual disabilities are at increased risk of both underweight and obesity, due to feeding problems such as dysphagia on one side and a sedentary lifestyle on the other; therefore a focus on nutrition status and healthy and balanced meal habits is crucial from an early age (Sullivan et al. 2000; Tanish et al. 2017).

Adults with disabilities often experience quantitative and qualitative inadequacy of diet and physical inactivity, resulting in a significant reduction of fat-free mass and bone mineral density. Despite their reduced muscle mass, a high percentage of adults with disabilities experience overweight. Several studies have shown that nutritional counselling alone seems to be ineffective and poorly applicable to people with disabilities (Krokstad et al. 2013). Body composition measurements can assist with monitoring changes in fat mass and skeletal muscle mass as the condition progresses.

When a person breathes, they lose moisture to the air each time they exhale – as much as two cups every day. In addition, a person's body loses water through evaporation from the surface of their skin even without demanding exercise. People also pass water through their urine. During the course of an average day, a healthy person may lose 8 to 10 glasses of water. When a person exercises, the amount of water they lose increases considerably. If people do not replace the water they lose through natural processes, they set off a physiological reaction that may have serious health effects. What follows is the natural progression of dehydration and the effects that has on the human body. To prevent dehydration, medical experts recommend that people drink at least 6 to 8 glasses of water every day as the best way to fight both the heat and cold (American College of Sports Medicine et al. 2016).

COMMON MEDICATIONS AND THEIR EFFECTS ON ASSESSMENT AND PHYSICAL ACTIVITY TOLERANCE

When creating an exercise programme it is important to understand the side effects of medications patients may be taking (American College of Sports Medicine et al. 2016). It may be necessary to make modifications to the warm-up and cool-down, the intensity of the programme, or how the intensity is monitored, the time of day at which you schedule a training session or class, etc. Making small adaptations such as these can allow for a programme to become more tailored, safe, and effective for the participants.

Some of the most common medications are:

Anti-convulsants are typically used to treat seizures. Epilepsy may be a primary diagnosis but is also common in CP (see Chapter 6). Common side effects may include dizziness, drowsiness, fatigue, nausea, tremor, rash, and weight gain.

Anti-spasticity/spasmolytics are muscle relaxants and are commonly used for individuals who have multiple sclerosis, spinal cord injury, CP, or who have had a stroke. The most common spasmolytic is Baclofen. Individuals using this medication may experience bradycardia (slow heart rate), hypotension (low blood pressure), sedation, dizziness, weakness, and/or discoordination, all of which have to be taken into account in the exercise programmes (see Chapters 6 and 8).

Beta blockers are commonly prescribed for individuals with cardiovascular disease. The most common exercise-related side effect of beta blockers is that they can severely reduce heart rate, and therefore they may cause a cap on the maximum heart rate. As a result, they may put restrictions on the person's exercise. Beta blockers are contraindicated in persons with asthma.

PRECAUTIONS AND ADAPTATIONS

Precautions and adaptations in the presence of:

Asthma

One of the most common respiratory disorders in childhood is asthma, which can lead to significant limitation in physical activity. Several factors like cold air or environmental pollutants may trigger or worsen the symptoms. Exercise-induced asthma is a narrowing of the airways in the lungs that is triggered by strenuous exercise. It causes shortness of breath, wheezing, coughing, and other symptoms during or after exercise. Swimming has been recognized as being less likely to cause symptoms of asthma than land-based activities due to the warmer, more humid environment. Treatment with common asthma medications and preventive measures enable people with asthma to exercise and remain active.

Congenital Heart Disease

Most children have surgical repair of the defect, and the aim of the treatment is the ability to lead a normal life. There is often need for tailored cardiac rehabilitation programmes that may improve exercise performance and reduce morbidity. Later on, recommendations are based on the severity of the heart condition. Those who have undergone successful surgery with minimal or no symptoms can lead a physically normal and active lifestyle. People with more severe and complicated conditions should still be encouraged to be physically active, but the intensity of the sports and exercises must be adapted, and strenuous forms should be avoided. It is complicated to establish an intensity threshold for aerobic training in patients with congenital heart diseases. Most often lactate measurements, percentage of peak heart rate, or percentage of peak work load are used, but so far no training intensity threshold for patients with congenital heart diseases has been identified.

Epilepsy

Almost all persons with epilepsy, both children and adults, are on medication, so the side effects of these medications have to be taken into account. It is important to have available acute medication for the treatment of unexpected seizures. People with epilepsy can safely participate in many physical activities. Regular exercise and physical activity are encouraged, as people with epilepsy achieve the same benefits from regular physical activity as people without epilepsy. It is important to stay hydrated and to ensure the participants have eaten a nutritious meal before exercise to help maintain blood sugar levels. One should wear protective gear associated with the activity (i.e. a helmet when cycling or roller-skating, etc.). There are different types of epilepsy and those who experience sudden seizures without a warning (aura) should avoid activities that are associated with a risk of falling or drowning.

Visual and Hearing Impairments

People with visual or hearing impairments have the capacity to enjoy a host of activities, with the assistance, as needed, of necessary adaptations and support systems. There are no contraindications to take part in any activity they prefer. Children with these impairments should be introduced to all sports, games, and activities that their peers learn. Lifetime activities such as tandem cycling, running, playing football, swimming, skiing, and bowling should be included as well. Not having access to these activities may result in children with these impairments not developing lifelong movement (or social) skills. They become adults who are unable to enjoy basic movement opportunities and who remain inactive over the life span.

Osteoarthritis

Exercise is considered the most effective non-drug treatment for reducing pain and improving movement in osteoarthritis. Three types of exercise are important for people with osteoarthritis: exercises involving range of motion, also called flexibility exercises; endurance or aerobic exercises; and strengthening exercises. Injuries like falls or severe bangs during athletic activities can cause major damage to the cartilage. It is important to avoid these kinds of injuries. Warming up and stretching before athletic activity and exercise can help prevent serious injury. Many adults with arthritis are inactive, and the first key to starting activity safely is to start gently; the second key is to go slow. Chapter 2 describes useful measurements and general training principles.

Osteoporosis

Osteoporosis is characterized by the loss of calcium in a person's bones, which makes them more at risk of fracture. Exercising regularly reduces the rate of bone loss and conserves bone tissue, thus lowering the risk of fractures. Physical activity is beneficial for bone mass, muscle strength, balance performance, and pain relief; exercise also helps reduce the risk of falling. Persons with osteoporosis need adequate and skilled supervision for their individual rehabilitation and training. They should avoid activities that involve loaded forward flexion of the spine such as abdominal sit-ups, or that require sudden forceful movement, unless introduced gradually as part of a progressive programme. Movements that require a forceful twisting motion, such as a golf swing, should also be avoided unless the person is accustomed to such movements and activities that carry a risk of falling.

Hypertension and Type 2 Diabetes

Both these conditions are frequently occurring medical entities but are not particularly typical for this group of children and adults with impaired functioning.

Spasticity and Dyskinesia

Both are symptoms frequently seen in CP (see Chapter 6) but also in a variety of neurological conditions. The main aims of physical therapy and training for people with these conditions are to reduce muscle tone, increase strength and coordination, and maintain or improve range of motion. The restorative nature of these measures is important to have in mind since intensity or duration that is too high can cause injury or unnecessary pain.

SPECIFIC RECOMMENDATIONS FOR EXERCISE PRE-PARTICIPATION HEALTH SCREENING

The American College of Sports Medicines' (ACSM) exercise pre-participation health screening process is aimed at identifying individuals with an elevated risk for exercise-related sudden cardiac death and/or acute myocardial infarction (American College of Sports Medicine et al. 2014). However, a scientific round table consensus at the ACSM conference in 2014 agreed that the existing exercise pre-participation health screening guidelines could result in excessive physician referrals and potentially reduce exercise participation (Riebe et al. 2015). There is also comprehensive evidence that exercise is not only safe for most people but has many health and fitness benefits (Garber et al.

2011; American College of Sports Medicine et al. 2016). Cardiovascular events are often preceded by warning signs or symptoms and the cardiovascular risks lessen with more physical activity and fitness (Bauman et al. 2002; Franklin and Billecke 2012; Fletcher et al. 2013; American College of Sports Medicine et al. 2016).

A new evidence-informed model for exercise pre-participation health screening was published based on three identified risk modulators: (1) the individual's current level of physical activity, (2) presence of signs or symptoms and/or known cardiovascular, metabolic, or renal disease, and (3) desired exercise intensity (Riebe et al. 2015). Identifying cardiovascular disease risk factors is still important, but risk factor profiling is not considered necessary in the exercise pre-participation health screening. These new ACSM recommendations reduce potential unnecessary barriers to a regular exercise programme and habitual physical activity, and thereby emphasize the importance of regular physical activity for all individuals (Riebe et al. 2015).

The new exercise pre-participation health screening guidelines are based on current levels of regular physical activity, major signs, or symptoms that indicate cardiovascular, metabolic, or renal diseases, and preferred exercise intensity. After the determination of the physical activity participation level (defined as regular, moderately intensive physical activity for at least 30 minutes for 3 days/week or more for the last 3 months or more), the participants are placed into the 'no' branch to the left, or the 'yes' branch on the right side (American College of Sports Medicine et al. 2014).

Guidelines for individuals who are currently active (American College of Sports Medicine et al. 2014; Riebe et al. 2015):

1. If they have no known cardiovascular, metabolic, or renal diseases, they may continue their exercise programme and progress gradually according to the ACSM guidelines.
2. If they have no known cardiovascular, metabolic, or renal diseases during the last 12 months, the exercise programme may be continued as long as the participants remain symptom free.
3. If symptoms occur, with or without known cardiovascular, metabolic, or renal diseases, the participants should stop the exercise programme until medical clearance is given.

Guidelines for individuals who are currently inactive (American College of Sports Medicine et al. 2014; Riebe et al. 2015):

1. If they have no known cardiovascular, metabolic, or renal diseases, they may participate in a light to moderate intensity exercise programme and progress gradually according to the ACSM guidelines.
2. If they have no symptoms but known cardiovascular, metabolic, or renal diseases, they should not start a new exercise programme until medical clearance is given.

3. If they have symptoms, with or without known cardiovascular, metabolic, or renal diseases, they should not start a new exercise programme until medical clearance is given.

SPECIFIC CONSIDERATIONS FOR CHILDREN

The World Health Organization recommends that children and adolescents aged 5 to 17 years should do at least 60 minutes of moderate- to vigorous-intensity physical activity every day, including activities that strengthen muscle and bone, at least three times per week (World Health Organization 2010; World Health Organization 2022). These recommendations underline the need for health care providers and physical education teachers to develop well-designed and integrated types of strength and conditioning into safe, age-appropriate, effective, and enjoyable programmes (Myer et al. 2011) (see Chapter 2). Many children and adolescents participate in sports, and some sports start with competitions at an early age. This may give cumulative workload, and therefore it is important to establish guidelines for age-appropriate training to enhance participation in physical activity without increasing the risk of sports-related injury. The cumulative workload has to be taken into consideration and incorporated into age-appropriate guidelines to prevent injuries, as sports and overexertion are the most common causes of all injury-related visits to primary care physicians by children and adolescents (Hambidge et al. 2002).

Integrative training combines health- and skill-related components of physical fitness into a programme with both specific strength and conditioning activities. Five key components of integrative training are underscored by Myer et al. (2011):

1. Age-appropriate education and instruction by qualified professionals who understand the physical and psychosocial uniqueness of children and adolescents. Two-thirds of strength training-related injuries in children are caused by accidents such as weights falling on the person, while sprains and strains are more common with increasing age (Myer et al. 2009). This points to the need for qualified instructors and a safe environment for such training, and children should be old enough to understand and follow instructions; 7 to 8 years is recommended as a starting age.

2. Mastery of fundamental movement skills is also required to prevent non-accidental injuries and to be able to follow instructions.

3. Gradual progression of training programmes should be emphasized. Regular progressive and multifaceted resistance training may contribute to reducing the risk of injury by the beneficial adaptations in bones, ligaments, and tendons following training. These adaptations from pre-season and in-season training programmes are shown to reduce the prevalence of injuries, e.g. in football players (Lehnhard et al. 1996).

4. Exercise variation is important to avoid strain on certain parts of the body. The selected exercises must be adapted to the individual participant's body size, fitness

level, exercise technique, and interests. For instance, children and young people can strengthen their core musculature without the aid of external resistance safely and effectively. Combined with balance training this will contribute to prevention of strain injuries.

5. A progressive conditioning programme integrating resistance, power, and speed training with periodic change of training volume and intensity throughout the year is recommended. Adequate recovery between challenging training sessions is very important but is sometimes overlooked in children. Integrative training programmes for any age group involve balancing training with recovery, which are both parts of individual adaptation. The instructors should be aware of the symptoms of over-training, such as long-lasting muscle soreness, decrease in performance, and reduced training motivation, and should be aware that children with variable maturity regarding musculoskeletal systems may not have the same exercise toleration as their peers without disability.

Several risk factors associated with strength training and conditioning for children and young people are modifiable by provision of qualified professionals (Faigenbaum et al. 2011). Lack of supervision is a risk factor that could be eliminated by substantive and timely instruction in adequate training spaces, where there are clear safety rules and where exercise equipment is stored securely. Clear instruction and feedback on exercise movements combined with prescribed progression programmes are important to avoid excessive load and volume, which can cause overload and injuries. Goal-directed and targeted training is important, in addition to adequate nutrition and balance between activity and rest to achieve optimal recovery (Faigenbaum et al. 2011).

REFERENCES

American College of Sports Medicine, Moore G, Durstine JL, Painter P (2016) *ACSM's Exercise Management for Persons with Chronic Diseases and Disabilities.* Champaign, IL: Human Kinetics.

American College of Sports Medicine, Pescatello LS, Arena R, Riebe D, Thompson PD, editors (2014) *ACSM's Guidelines for Exercise Testing and Prescription,* 9th ed. Philadelphia, PA: Wolters Kluwer/Lippincott Williams & Wilkins Health.

Bauman AE, Sallis JF, Dzewaltowski DA, Owen N (2002) Toward a better understanding of the influences on physical activity: the role of determinants, correlates, causal variables, mediators, moderators, and confounders. *Am J Prev Med* **23**: 5–14.

Felleskatalogen AS I (2017) *The Norwegian Pharmaceutical Product Compendium* [online]. Available at: https://www.felleskatalogen.no/medisin [Accessed 4 October 2022].

Fletcher GF, Ades PA, Kligfield P et al. (2013) Exercise standards for testing and training: a scientific statement from the American Heart Association. *Circulation* **128**: 873–934.

Franklin BA, Billecke S (2012) Putting the benefits and risks of aerobic exercise in perspective. *Curr Sports Med Rep* **11**(4): 201–208.

Garber CE, Blissmer B, Deschenes MR et al. (2011) American College of Sports Medicine position stand. Quantity and quality of exercise for developing and maintaining cardiorespiratory, musculoskeletal, and neuromotor fitness in apparently healthy adults: guidance for prescribing exercise. *Med Sci Sports Exerc* **43**: 1334–1359. Special communication. 10.1249/MSS.0b013e318213fefb.

Goodman JM, Thomas SG, Burr J (2011) Evidence-based risk assessment and recommendations for exercise testing and physical activity clearance in apparently healthy individuals. *Appl Physiol Nutr Metab* **36**: S14–32.

Hadden KL, von Baeyer CL (2002) Pain in children with cerebral palsy: common triggers and expressive behaviors. *Pain* **99**: 281–288.

Hambidge SJ, Davidson AJ, Gonzales R, Steiner JF (2002) Epidemiology of pediatric injury-related primary care office visits in the United States. *Pediatrics* **109**: 559–565.

Jahnsen R, Villien L, Aamodt G, Stanghelle JK, Holm I (2004) Musculoskeletal pain in adults with cerebral palsy compared with the general population. *Journal of Rehabilitation Medicine* **36**: 78–84.

IASP (2004) Pain Clinical Updates. *Neuropathic Pain: The Immune Connection.* International Association for the Study of Pain (IASP), 2004, Volume XII, No. 1.

Kohl HW 3rd, Craig CL, Lambert EV et al. (2012) The pandemic of physical inactivity: global action for public health. *Lancet* **380**: 294–305.

Krokstad S, Knudtsen MS, Hveem K et al. (2013) Cohort Profile: the HUNT Study, Norway. *Int J Epidemiol* **42**: 968–977.

Lehnhard RA, Lehnhard HR, Young R, Butterfield SA (1996) Monitoring injuries on a college soccer team: the effect of strength training. *J Strength Cond Res* **10**: 115–119.

Merkel SI, Voepel-Lewis T, Shayevitz JR, Malviya S (1997) The FLACC: a behavioral scale for scoring postoperative pain in young children. *Pediatr Nurs* **23**: 293–297.

Merskey H, Bogduk N eds (1994) *Classification of Chronic Pain: IASP Task Force on Taxonomy*, 2nd ed. Seattle: IASP Press.

Myer GD, Faigenbaum AD, Chu DA et al. (2011) Integrative training for children and adolescents: techniques and practices for reducing sports-related injuries and enhancing athletic performance. *The Physician and Sportsmedicine* **39**: 74–84. 10.3810/psm.2011.02.1864.

Myer GD, Quatman CE, Khoury J, Wall EJ, Hewett TE (2009) Youth versus adult 'weightlifting' injuries presenting to United States emergency rooms: accidental versus non-accidental injury mechanisms. *J Strength Cond Res* **23**: 2054–2060.

Ramstad K, Jahnsen R, Skjeldal OH, Diseth TH (2011) Characteristics of recurrent musculoskeletal pain in children with cerebral palsy aged 8 to 18 years. *Dev Med Child Neurol* **53**: 1013–1018.

Riebe D, Franklin BA, Thompson PD et al. (2015) Updating ACSM's recommendations for exercise preparticipation health screening. *Medicine & Science in Sports & Exercise* **47**: 2473–2479. 10.1249/MSS.0000000000000664.

Russo RN, Miller MD, Haan E, Cameron ID, Crotty M (2008) Pain characteristics and their association with quality of life and self-concept in children with hemiplegic cerebral palsy identified from a population register. *Clin J Pain* **24**: 335–342.

Sullivan PB, Lambert B, Rose M, Ford-Adams M, Johnson A, Griffiths P (2000) Prevalence and severity of feeding and nutritional problems in children with neurological impairment: Oxford Feeding Study. *Dev Med Child Neurol* **42**: 674–680.

Tanish HI, Curtin C, Must A, Phillips S, Maslin M, Bandini LG (2017) Physical Activity levels, frequency, and type among adolescents with and without autism spectrum disorder. *J Autism Dev Disord* **47**: 785–794.

Tomlinson D, von Baeyer CL, Stinson JN, Sung L (2010) A systematic review of faces scales for the self-report of pain intensity in children. *Pediatrics* **126**: e1168-98. 10.1542/peds. 2010-1609.

World Health Organization (2010) *Global Recommendations on Physical Activity for Health* [online]. Available at: https://www.who.int/publications/i/item/9789241599979 [Accessed 1 January 2010].

World Health Organization (2022) *Physical Activity*. Fact sheet [online]. Updated February 2017. Available at: http://www.who.int/mediacentre/factsheets/fs385/en/ [Accessed 5 October 2022].

Wong DL, Baker CM (1988) Pain in children: comparison of assessment scales. *Pediatric Nursing* **14**: 9–17.

CHAPTER 4

Principles of Measuring Physical Activity

Carol Maher and Dot Dumuid

INTRODUCTION

Physical activity has been described as any bodily movement produced by skeletal muscles that results in a substantial increase over resting energy expenditure (Bouchard and Shepard 1994). The health benefits of physical activity are wide and varied. In adults, the health effects of physical activity include reduced risk of coronary heart disease, hypertension, type 2 diabetes, obesity, certain cancers, and some mental health problems (Haskell et al. 2007). Long-term prospective studies have shown that the risk of mortality is significantly lower in physically active and/or fit adults compared with their inactive counterparts, and that mid-life increases in physical activity or fitness are associated with significant reductions in risk of mortality (Haskell et al. 2007). Since chronic health conditions such as heart disease, stroke, and diabetes are far less common in childhood, the effect of physical activity on morbidity and mortality in children and adolescents is less clear. However, evidence suggests that physical activity contributes to optimal health and well-being in children and adolescents, including cardiovascular health, maintenance of healthy weight, improved bone density, and improved psychological health (Janssen and LeBlanc 2010). Among children and adults with physical disabilities, physical activity appears to hold additional benefits in terms of maximizing and maintaining functional ability and independence with activities of daily living.

Physical activity encompasses activities undertaken in a wide variety of contexts, such as active leisure, sport, exercise, occupational activity, chores, and active transport (e.g. walking and cycling). It can vary in terms of timing (e.g. the duration of the physical activity and whether it is undertaken in several intermittent bouts versus a single continuous bout) and intensity. In general, the strongest benefits are associated with moderate-to-vigorous physical activity, which can be loosely defined as brisk walking and above, or activity of sufficient intensity to cause moderate puffing. There is emerging evidence that light-intensity activity may hold some benefit.

In order for individuals, clinicians, and researchers to understand the physical activity requirement of children and adults with physical disabilities, plan services, and evaluate the impact of services, accurate tools for measuring physical activity are required.

TYPES OF PHYSICAL ACTIVITY MEASURES

A wide variety of physical activity measurement tools are available. However, there is no single standout 'best' measurement tool; each tool possesses advantages and disadvantages. Some tools must be undertaken under laboratory settings, and others are designed for free-living conditions (Fig. 4.1).

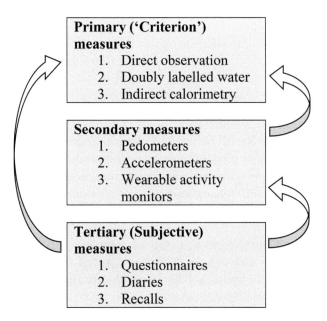

Figure 4.1 Physical activity measurement methods can classified into three hierarchical categories: primary, secondary, and tertiary. The arrows indicate commonly acceptable criterion standards for the validation of secondary and tertiary measures; i.e. a secondary measure is ideally validated against a primary measure, while a tertiary measure can be validated against either a secondary or a primary measure. The primary and secondary measures listed are objective, and so are often considered to be more scientifically rigorous, because they are free of subjective sources of bias, such as recall and social desirability bias. However, the primary and secondary measures are unable to capture contextual aspects of physical activity, such as the location or type of physical activity undertaken (with the exception of direct observation). For this reason, it is common for tertiary (subjective) measures of physical activity to be used in combination with objective measures

This means the choice of tool may depend upon the setting as well as what is available in terms of tools and the expertise to use them. This chapter provides an overview of key physical activity measurement methodologies. This includes a discussion of the tools' reliability (the extent to which the tool can secure consistent results) and validity (how well the tool truly measures what it sets out to measure) in both general child and adult populations, and wherever possible, in children and adults with physical disabilities. The chapter will consider pertinent practical issues regarding the selection and application of these measurement tools in a variety of self-monitoring, clinical, and research settings. Many of the measurement methods currently available are suited to ambulant children and adults with physical disabilities. A section at the end of the chapter will be devoted to measurement of physical activity in individuals who use wheelchairs to ambulate. Laboratory-based physical activity measurement techniques will be presented briefly; however, the focus of the chapter will be on lower cost and more pragmatic physical activity measurement options.

Primary and Laboratory Measures of Physical Activity

Two common laboratory-based measures of physical activity are doubly labelled water and calorimetry. The **doubly labelled water technique** measures total energy expenditure over a 1- to 2-week period. Participants drink water containing 'labelled' isotopes of oxygen and hydrogen. Over the next 5 to 14 days the labelled hydrogen is eliminated from the body as water, and the labelled oxygen is eliminated as water and carbon dioxide. The amount of the labelled isotopes left in the body is determined from periodic urine samples, and the total energy expenditure is calculated from the difference in elimination rates (Park et al. 2014). Advantages of the doubly labelled water technique are that it is objective, has low reactivity (i.e. there is relatively low chance that a participant will change their activities as a result of being measured), has well-established reliability and validity, and is non-obtrusive. However, doubly labelled water is very expensive, in terms of the labelled water itself, stringent administration protocols involved, and the need for highly specialized laboratory analysis. In addition, doubly labelled water does not provide any information on how the energy was expended (activity, frequency, intensity, duration).

Indirect calorimetry measures energy expenditure by measuring a participant's oxygen consumption and carbon dioxide production via a face mask, a hood, or within a respiratory chamber, which is a sealed room set up in a laboratory designed to simulate a free-living room. Indirect calorimetry is considered a valid and accurate measure of physical activity (Psota and Chen 2013) and is used extensively. Disadvantages of indirect calorimetry are that it requires gas analysis equipment, so tends to be used in laboratory or contrived settings as opposed to free-living conditions. For example, indirect calorimetry can be undertaken over a long duration (e.g. 24 hours) within a respiratory chamber; however, this does not provide accurate information on activities of daily living in free-living conditions. Indirect calorimetry can also be undertaken using a portable system with a face mask or hood to measure specific free-living activities over a short duration (e.g. 10–20 min). For example, indirect calorimetry can be used to evaluate whether orthopaedic surgery leads to a more energy-efficient gait pattern. However, the technique requires strict adherence to a protocol such as fasting and remaining at rest before and during measurement, and children may become restless during the evaluation period. Furthermore, children with disabilities may be particularly sensitive to wearing a face mask (Trost and O'Neill 2013).

Direct observation involves an observer recording the frequency, duration, and intensity of a participant's activity. Since it involves direct measurement of physical activity, it is often considered a 'primary' measurement technique. Numerous standardized techniques have been developed to enhance the reliability of direct observation, including the Observational System for Recording Physical Activity in Children (McIver et al. 2016) and the System for Observing Fitness Instruction Time (Rowe et al. 1997). In many ways, direct observation is the best physical activity behaviour measurement (Trost 2007). It has the advantage of being able to capture the type of activity performed, as well as environmental conditions, social context, and the use of assistive equipment. Direct observation can be particularly useful for populations with physical disabilities, as observers are able to distinguish between sedentary and physically active tasks, which may not be achieved by instruments such as pedometers due to irregular movement patterns. However, direct observation is time-intensive, limiting its large-scale use (Corder et al. 2008). Additionally, observers require extensive training to improve intra- and inter-rater reliability and participants may change their behaviour in reaction to being observed (Sirard and Pate 2001).

Secondary Physical Activity Measures

Secondary physical activity instruments include wearable devices that provide objective assessment of the amount of physical activity. At their most basic, secondary physical activity measurement tools can capture one metric of physical activity (e.g. pedometers, which measure steps), while more advanced secondary physical activity measurement tools, such as accelerometers, can capture numerous aspects of physical activity, such as frequency, intensity, and duration of activity. However, secondary instruments are unable to capture the type of activity, location, or context. Secondary objective measures are obtained from devices attached to the participant's body at a specific location. Traditionally, pedometers and accelerometers are worn on the waist, in line with the knee of the dominant leg (Silcott et al. 2011). However, with improvements in technology and user preferences, accelerometers are increasingly located on the wrist. Wrist-worn accelerometers are generally considered to have acceptable, albeit slightly lower, reliability and validity relative to waist-worn accelerometers, but they have demonstrated higher acceptability for wearers, resulting in improved wear-time compliance rates, particularly if a 24-hour wear-protocol is desired (Tudor Locke et al. 2015).

Device location requires special consideration among people with physical disabilities, as the presence of a limp or other movement disorder may influence the function of the device (Horvath et al. 2007). Location of the device nearer the wearer's centre of mass may provide more accurate estimations, as erroneous movements (e.g. jerky movement of the limbs) are less likely to be registered as activity counts. For people with unilateral impairment (e.g. unilateral cerebral palsy), the device should be located on the non-affected side. It is prudent to test the function of the device (e.g. a pedometer) in a variety of body locations, in order to determine the optimum location by comparing pedometer steps against manually counted steps.

PEDOMETERS

Pedometers are small, relatively inexpensive devices used to record the total number of steps taken in a given period of time. Numerous studies have validated pedometers against other measures of physical activity, including direct observation, accelerometry, and heart rate monitoring. Taken together, results suggest that pedometers have moderate to strong validity for measurement of physical activity, though validity varies between models of pedometers, and it is common for pedometers to underestimate step counts in free-living conditions (Silcott et al. 2011).

Pedometers often use algorithms to estimate distance travelled and energy expenditure; however, these outputs can have a high degree of error, so it is preferable to focus on steps. Most pedometers only capture the total number of steps in a given period (e.g. 24h or until manually reset), with no additional information regarding the intensity, duration, or frequency of activity (Corder et al. 2008). Consequently, steps accumulated during light and moderate intensity activities such as walking are recorded the same as those accumulated through vigorous activities such as running or stair climbing. In their most common position at the hip, pedometers do not register upper limb activities, such as carrying a load or pushing, or certain lower limb activities, such as cycling. A practical difficulty of using activity monitors with children and adolescent populations is the high rate of participants tampering with the monitors (Warren et al. 2010). This may be averted by using tape to hide the pedometer display from view.

Pedometers have been established as valid for use in people with physical disabilities. A systematic review of seven studies found the correlation between pedometer step counts and directly observed step counts in populations with physical disabilities was moderate to excellent (Kenyon et al. 2013). This suggests that the reliability and validity of pedometers in populations with physical disabilities is slightly lower than what is seen in the general population but still acceptable (Kenyon et al. 2013). A study examining the use of pedometers in 17 children with physical disabilities suggested that reliability and validity improve as the speed of locomotion increases (Maher et al. 2013).

Accelerometers

Accelerometers are small, relatively sophisticated electronic devices that record accelerations produced by body movement. In research settings, they have become the most commonly used objective measure of physical activity across all age groups (Cain et al. 2013). Many brands and models are available, with common examples including the Actigraph (Actigraph, Pensacola, FL, USA), Geneactiv (Activinsights Ltd, Kimbolton, UK), and ActivPAL (PAL Technologies, Glasgow, UK). Accelerometers have an internal clock and record the amount of acceleration ('counts') per pre-determined period of time ('epoch') set by the researcher, typically 1 minute (Cain et al. 2013). Higher activity counts represent higher physical activity intensity levels.

After use, the accelerometer data are downloaded to a computer, using a specialized dock or cable and software (Fig. 4.2). The software allows the accelerometer data to be collapsed and analysed into meaningful outputs, such as total number of counts per day, average counts per minute, and number of minutes of physical activity. Selecting appropriate count thresholds, or cut points, is essential for accurate estimation of physical activity levels. A wide variety of cut points have been proposed by different research

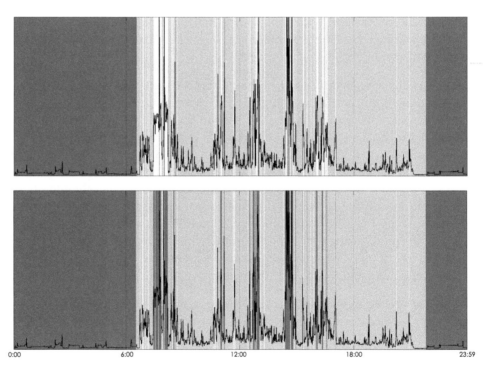

Figure 4.2 Example accelerometer trace for 24 hours of accelerometry data. Dark grey shading indicates sleep; light grey shading awake time. The trace indicates the magnitude of accelerations, with dark lines indicating periods of vigorous physical activity and light lines indicating periods of moderate physical activity

groups to differentiate moderate and vigorous physical activity, and estimates of daily physical activity can differ dramatically depending on which cut points are applied (up to around 400% difference [Corder et al. 2008]).

Numerous studies have validated accelerometers against other measures of physical activity, including doubly labelled water, indirect calorimetry, heart rate monitoring, and other makes and models of accelerometers. Studies generally show that validity of accelerometers is moderate-to-strong, and is gradually improving due to advancements in accelerometer technology.

Advantages of accelerometers are that they are easy to use in free-living conditions, do not interfere with participants' movement patterns, and can provide information on activity patterns. Most modern accelerometers do not have external controls, which minimizes the risk of tampering. Disadvantages include that accelerometry is expensive, in terms of equipment costs (devices typically cost >$200USD), and labour for preparing and processing the data. Also, accelerometers can underestimate physical activity, since the count for any given epoch is the average count, and thus if the participant moves vigorously and rests within the epoch, credit will not be given for having engaged in vigorous physical activity. Like pedometers, depending on device placement, accelerometers can be insensitive to certain forms of activity; for example, a hip-placed accelerometer will be insensitive to cycling and stair climbing. Also, accelerometers are generally not worn during water activities and contact sports (Knowlden 2015).

A systematic review of physical activity instruments used in children and young people with physical disabilities (White et al. 2016) found that accelerometers are the most commonly used objective measurement approach. Results of the review suggest that reliability and validity of accelerometers in young people with physical disabilities are good to excellent. It is important to note that cut points used for determining physical activity intensity in children and adults without disabilities may not be appropriate for children and adults with physical disabilities. Modified cut points have been validated for various age groups with cerebral palsy (Keawutan et al. 2016); however, these cut points should not be generalized to other disability groups (White et al. 2016).

Activity Trackers

In the early 2000s, accelerometer-based wearable devices were predominantly used in research and military contexts. However, as the technology has become smaller and cheaper, the field of consumer wearables has emerged and grown rapidly. Popular examples include Fitbits, Garmin, and the Apple watch, among others. These devices are typically worn on the wrist (or, less commonly, on the hip, chest, or neck) and capture daily movement using in-built accelerometers. The devices provide feedback on a wide range of physical activity metrics, such as daily step counts, moderate-to-vigorous physical activity minutes, energy expenditure, and stairs climbed, as well as sedentary time and sleep quality and quantity. Many wearable devices have a screen on the device itself that provides real-time feedback to the wearer. In addition, they use Bluetooth to transfer data wirelessly to a smartphone. Free, proprietary software can then be used to view activity data, typically in more detail than can be seen on the device itself.

Activity trackers have rapidly become popular personal devices that children and adults alike use to monitor and increase their physical activity. In clinical and research settings, activity trackers are also increasingly being used as an outcome measure to assess the impact of clinical interventions and programmes (such as activity levels before and after surgery). In these applications, activity trackers are essentially being used in place of research-oriented accelerometers, due to their lower costs and their user-friendly software interface, which makes data collection and processing more convenient for clinical and research personnel. However, activity trackers have some disadvantages for physical activity measurement. Most importantly, by design, wearable activity trackers are *intervention* tools, aimed at helping wearers increase their physical activity by providing detailed feedback and prompts to move. Thus, the risk of reactivity is high. Second, the activity data captured by activity trackers are automatically processed using proprietary algorithms that provide estimates of steps, physical activity level, and energy expenditure. These algorithms are fixed and lack transparency, unlike research-grade accelerometers, where the researcher or clinician has access to the raw accelerometry data, and the ability to choose from several validated algorithms to quantify physical activity depending on the participant population (e.g. toddlers, preschoolers, children and adolescents, and adults). Third, and related to this, the way that consumer activity trackers measure and provide feedback on physical activity can change when the manufacturers update their software and firmware. Indeed, Fitbit changed their algorithm for defining moderate to vigorous physical activity in 2015, and researchers have reported major software interface changes occurring mid-trial leading to data loss (Ferguson et al. 2015). To provide context, with moderate physical activity, breathing would be apparent, and the person could talk but not sing. With vigorous physical activity it would even be difficult to talk without pausing to take a breath. In typically developing child and adult populations, numerous studies have been conducted examining reliability and validity of a large variety of activity tracker models. Generally, studies evaluating trackers' reliability and validity report excellent validity for measurement of step counts (Evenson et al. 2015; Gorzelitz et al. 2020). Validity is slightly lower for other physical activity metrics (e.g. there was moderate to excellent validity for energy expenditure and moderate to vigorous physical activity time) and varies by tracker brand and model (Gorzelitz et al. 2020). More recently, some studies have reported the validity of activity trackers in ambulant children with disabilities. One study examined the validity of one hip and one wrist-worn Fitbit device (Fitbit 'One' and Fitbit 'Flex', respectively) in children with cerebral palsy, suggesting that the hip-worn Fitbit was accurate for measuring steps (r=0.99) but the wrist-worn Fitbit was not (r=−0.03) (Sala et al. 2019). Similarly, a small study (*n*=10) of the validity of the wrist-worn Fitbit 'Charge' in children with mobility-related disabilities found that validity was poor (Javorina 2020).

Tertiary Physical Activity Measures

Tertiary physical activity measures refer to subjective measures such as questionnaires, recalls, and diaries. They may be completed by either self-report or proxy-report (i.e. a parent, teacher, or carer completing it on a participant's behalf). In both instances, administration methods can also vary between self-administration and interview-administration. In general, self-report has greater validity than proxy report (Telford et al. 2004), since proxy reporters may not have monitored the target child or adult constantly for the entire period in question. Therefore, proxy-report is generally reserved for young children, or participants with recall or comprehension difficulties. For example, among children without disabilities, it has been found that children aged under 10 years cannot recall their activities and the timeframes of activities accurately (Baranowski et al. 1984). Also, they can have difficulty conceptualizing physical activity: while they may understand that traditional sports and recreational activities constitute physical activity, they frequently cannot differentiate between sedentary and active tasks encountered in daily life (such as playing on a computer vs sweeping) (Trost et al. 2000). The validity of interviewer-administration is generally higher than self-administration (Corder et al. 2008). In any case, subjective measures of physical activity will be influenced by the perceptions and opinions of the participant and/or proxy reporter.

PHYSICAL ACTIVITY QUESTIONNAIRES

Questionnaires are the most common instruments used to examine physical activity in large populations. An enormous array of questionnaires exists that vary in terms of the dimensions of physical activity examined (e.g. mode of exercise, frequency, duration, and intensity), the recall time frame (ranging from a day up to a year) and how the data are analysed (e.g. as a rating, arbitrary activity score, estimate of energy expenditure, daily or weekly minutes of physical activity etc.). Many physical activity questionnaires focus on leisure activities, without accounting for physical activity undertaken in daily activities such as household chores or active transport.

Questionnaires are generally quick and easy to administer, relatively inexpensive, and unobtrusive and non-reactive (i.e. unlikely to induce changes in physical activity behaviour as a result of the measurement process) (Trost 2005). However, given that they involve self-report, recall, and estimation, careful attention must be paid to their reliability and validity.

In a review of 27 physical activity questionnaires used with children (Ridley 2005), reliability and validity varied widely, from poor through to excellent. This range in reliability and validity is likely to reflect both the quality of the instruments themselves (how well the questions are framed), and also the protocol that was used for evaluating reliability and validity. In general, instruments that seek to measure physical activity over an extended period of time (such as 6 months) tend to perform more poorly than instruments that measure physical activity over a shorter period (e.g. a week).

Few physical activity questionnaires have been specifically evaluated for use in physical disability populations. A 2016 systematic review (White et al. 2016) found that while numerous physical activity instruments have been used in paediatric physical disability populations, only two have been scrutinized for reliability and validity in disability populations. In terms of validity, Maher et al. (2007) found that the Physical Activity Questionnaire for Adolescents, originally created by Kowalski et al. (1997), had weak correlations with pedometry and accelerometry in children with cerebral palsy. Similarly, Takken et al. (2003) reported that their purpose-designed questionnaire showed weak correlation with accelerometry in children with juvenile arthritis. The questionnaires performed better in terms of reliability, with the Physical Activity Questionnaire for Adolescents having excellent reliability in children with cerebral palsy (Maher et al. 2007). In addition, the Activities Scale for Kids – performance version – has excellent reliability (Young et al. 2000); however, its validity has not been examined. Longmuir and Bar-Or (2000) reported a pilot study that examined the reliability of the Canada Fitness Survey among young people with disabilities and reported moderate to excellent reliability.

Clinicians and researchers seeking to measure physical activity using a questionnaire may find the process of selecting of an instrument bewildering. Careful attention should be paid to the questionnaire items and time frame to ensure that it captures the aspects of physical activity of interest. Additionally, evidence of reliability and validity should be considered.

Physical Activity Diaries

Physical activity diaries require participants to log all of their daily activities in predefined epochs (typically 15min increments), and are usually undertaken for a number of days. Diaries may be paper-based or computer-based, and some are linked to energy cost compendia, allowing estimation of energy expenditure. Advantages of diaries are that they reduce recall bias compared with other tertiary methods. However, disadvantages include high participant burden, high potential for reactivity, and lack of clarity (e.g. even 15-min epochs may be too long to capture many physical activities).

Few studies have evaluated the validity of self-report diaries in the child and adolescent populations. Rodriguez et al. (2002) compared total energy expenditure estimated from a 24-hour diary with total energy expenditure calculated from heart rate monitoring in a sample of 20 children, aged 5 to 16 years, and found a strong agreement between the two measurement methods. No studies have examined the validity of physical activity diaries in participants with physical disabilities.

Physical Activity Recalls

Physical activity recalls are similar to physical activity diaries, in that participants are required to report all of their daily activities in predefined epochs. However, unlike diaries that are completed prospectively, recalls are completed retrospectively (e.g. children are asked to recall the previous day). This reduces reactivity and burden but increases the potential for recall bias compared with diary methodologies. A 1-day computer-based recall, the Multimedia Activity Recall for Children and Adults (MARCA), has been shown to have excellent reliability in children and adults without disabilities and moderate validity relative to pedometry and accelerometry (Olds et al. 2010). However, among children and adolescents with cerebral palsy, the Multimedia Activity Recall for Children and Adults has only fair validity relative to pedometry (Maher 2008).

OTHER MEASUREMENT CONSIDERATIONS

Both children's and adults' physical activities vary from day to day, depending on lifestyle demands and leisure activities undertaken. In particular, it is well recognized that children's physical activity differs between school days and non-school days (as do adults' between weekdays and weekend days), and also according to the weather conditions and season. Given this, habitual or 'usual' physical activity is likely to be under- or over-estimated if only 1 day of activity is measured; thus it is usually recommended that physical activity is measured across a prolonged period, with particular attention paid to ensure that both weekday and weekend days are captured.

Questionnaires commonly account for this in their reference frame (e.g. they will commonly ask questions about physical activity in the 'past week' or 'past month'). For diaries and recalls (which typically measure physical activity across a 24-h period), multiple days of data are gathered. For example, the Multimedia Activity Recall for Children and Adults is typically collected for 4 days, and a range of day types is purposely sampled (i.e. at least 1 weekday and 1 weekend day). For objective continuous monitoring methods such as pedometry and accelerometry, it is common for 7 days of data to be collected. Minimum wear time rules are usually applied; for example, for a day of monitoring to be considered complete, researchers will commonly stipulate that device should have been worn for ≥10 waking hours. In fact, 24-hour wear-protocols are becoming increasingly common. This has two key advantages: first, it generally leads to the device being worn for more waking hours each day, and second, in the case of accelerometry, wearing the device during sleep can provide additional data regarding sleep duration and quality (Tudor Locke et al. 2015). At a minimum, studies should capture at least 4 full days of data, including 1 weekend day (Corder et al. 2008). Data can be used to calculate average weekly physical activity by weighting weekday and weekend day data 5:2.

Seasonal variables, such as school holidays and climate impact physical activity. Lewis et al. (2016) found that physical activity levels peak around 20°C to 25°C, and steadily decline at temperatures higher and lower than this. Additionally, rain reduces physical activity, whereas snow does not. Such variables should be taken into account where physical activity is being measured over a long period of time, such as in longitudinal studies.

MEASUREMENT OF PHYSICAL ACTIVITY IN WHEELCHAIR-AMBULANT CHILDREN

Measurement of physical activity amongst children who use a wheelchair to ambulate requires special consideration. Very few data exist regarding the reliability and validity of physical activity measurement methods for children and adults with physical disabilities who use a wheelchair. Given the lack of empirical evidence, face validity would suggest that direct observation is likely to be the most accurate form of measurement (Fig. 4.3). Where this is not feasible, self-reported measures, such as questionnaires, diaries, and recalls may be appropriate. Special attention should be paid to the suitability of the questionnaire items. In the case of diaries and recalls, energy expenditure estimates likely have unacceptably high error, due to the large differences in energy costs for completing comparable tasks (e.g. standing vs in a wheelchair).

In our experience, many children and adults who have physical disabilities that require them to use a wheelchair will typically have a powered wheelchair or are pushed in a

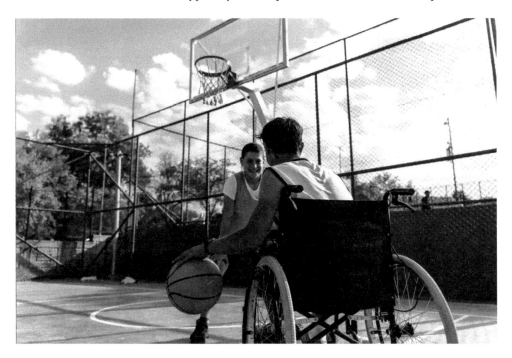

Figure 4.3 Measurement of physical activity in children who are wheelchair ambulant presents additional challenges. 'iStock.com/Phynart Studio'

manual wheelchair. In the case of children and adults with physical disabilities who self-propel in a manual wheelchair, objective physical activity measures such as pedometers or accelerometers may be useful. Nooijen et al. (2015) found that a five-point accelerometry array attached to children's sternum, wrists, and thighs was able to detect physical activity with high accuracy compared to direct observation. However, this set-up is impractical for free-living contexts and is only likely to be useful in research applications. Another study reported a protocol in which an accelerometer was mounted directly on the manual wheelchair. When evaluated with adult participants without disabilities, they reported excellent accuracy for detecting physical activity involved with propulsion and activities of daily living.

The key features, strengths, and limitations of physical activity measurement methods for people with physical disabilities are summarized in Table 4.1.

KEY POINTS FOR MEASUREMENT OF PHYSICAL ACTIVITY AMONG PEOPLE WITH PHYSICAL DISABILITIES

A multitude of methods are available to measure physical activity, and these may be classified into primary, secondary, or tertiary measures.

Selection of the most appropriate method will depend on:
• The clinical or research question being addressed, as outlined below;
• The type of physical activity of interest (e.g. recording total energy expenditure vs needing to record characteristics such as the frequency, duration, and intensity of an activity);
• The duration of the activity (e.g. studying a discrete physical activity, vs studying habitual physical activity in free-living conditions);
• The number of participants involved;
• The budget;
• Participants' characteristics (e.g. age, cognitive ability, form of ambulation, and acceptable level of participation burden).

There is limited evidence confirming the reliability and validity of physical activity measurement methods for use specifically with people with disabilities. In general, the validity of physical activity measurement tools tends to be slightly lower when used with people with disabilities compared with the same tool used with people without disabilities. Regardless, a number of tools have acceptable validity. The ability to measure physical activity accurately is important in order to understand the physical activity levels and characteristics among people with physical disabilities, and to measure the impact of clinical interventions and physical activity programmes designed to improve fitness.

Table 4.1 Key attributes of physical activity measurement methods

Method	Valid	Cheap	Objective	Ease of administration	Easy to complete	Measures patterns, modes, and dimensions of physical activity	Non-reactive*	Feasible in large studies	Suitability for ages <10 years or cognitive impairment	Suitable for wheelchair ambulant individuals
Primary measures										
Direct observation	+++	-	++	+	+++	++	+	+	+++	+++
Doubly labelled water	+++	-	+++	++	++	-	++	-	++	+++
Indirect calorimetry	+++	-	+++	+	+	-	+	-	+	+
Secondary measures										
Pedometer	++	+++	+++	++	++	-	+	+++	+++	+ self-prop only
Accelerometer	++	+	+++	++	++	++	++	++	+++	+ self-prop only
Activity monitors	++	++	+++	++	++	++	-	++	+++	+ self-prop only
Tertiary measures										
Questionnaire	+	+++	-	+++	++	+++	+++	+++	++ proxy	+
Diary	++	+++	-	+++	-	+++	-	+	++ proxy	+
Recall	++	+++	-	+++	+	+++	+	+	++ proxy	+

+++ Excellent
++ Good
+ Acceptable
- Poor or inappropriate
* Non-reactive – unlikely to induce changes in physical activity behaviour as a result of the measurement process

REFERENCES

Baranowski T, Dworkin R, Cieslik C et al. (1984) Reliability and validity of self-report of aerobic activity: family health project. *Research Quarterly for Exercise and Sport* **55**: 309–317.

Bouchard C, Shepard RJ (1994) Physical activity, fitness and health: the model and key concepts. In: Bouchard C, Shepard RJ, Stephens T, editors, *Physical Activity, Fitness and Health.* Champaign, IL: Human Kinetics, pp 77–88.

Cain K, Sallis J, Conway T, Van Dyck D, Calhoon L (2013) Using accelerometers in youth physical activity studies: a review of methods. *Journal of Physical Activity and Health* **10**: 437–450.

Corder K, Ekelund U, Steele R, Wareham N, Brage S (2008) Assessment of physical activity in youth. *Journal of Applied Physiology* **105**: 977–987.

Evenson K, Goto M, Furberg R (2015) Systematic review of the validity and reliability of consumer-wearable activity trackers. *International Journal of Behavioral Nutrition and Physical Activity* **12**: 159.

Ferguson T, Rowlands A, Olds T, Maher C (2015) The validity of consumer-level, activity monitors in healthy adults worn in free-living conditions: a cross-sectional study. *International Journal of Behavioral Nutrition and Physical Activity* **12**: 42.

Gorzelitz J, Farber C, Gangnon R, Cadmus-Bertram L (2020) Accuracy of wearable trackers for measuring moderate-to vigorous-intensity physical activity: a systematic review and meta-analysis. *Journal for the Measurement of Physical Behaviour* **3**: 346–357.

Haskell WL, Lee I-M, Pate RR et al. (2007) Physical activity and public health: updated recommendation for adults from the American College of Sports Medicine and the American Heart Association. *Circulation* **116**: 1081.

Horvath S, Taylor D, Marsh J, Kriellaarsa D (2007) The effect of pedometer position and normal gait asymmetry on step count accuracy: found axillary position to be most accurate. *Applied Physiology, Nutrition, and Metabolism* **32**: 409–415.

Janssen I, Leblanc AG (2010) Systematic review of the health benefits of physical activity and fitness in school-aged children and youth. *International Journal of Behavioral Nutrition and Physical Activity* **7**: 40.

Javorina D (2020) *Investigating the Validity of the Fitbit ChargeHR TM for Measuring Physical Activity in Children and Youth with Mobility-Related Disabilities.* Master's thesis, University of Toronto.

Keawutan P, Bell K, Oftedal S, Davies P, Boyd R (2016) Validation of accelerometer cut-points in children with cerebral palsy aged 4 to 5 years. *Pediatric Physical Therapy* **28**: 427–434.

Kenyon A, McEvoy M, Sprod J, Maher C (2013) Validity of pedometers in people with physical disabilities: a systematic review. *Archives of Physical Medicine and Rehabilitation* **94**: 1161–1170.

Knowlden A (2015) Measurement of physical activity for health promotion and education research. *Arch Exerc Health Dis* **5**: 338–345.

Kowalski K, Crocker P, Faulkner R (1997) Validation of the physical activity questionnaire for older children. *Pediatric Exercise Science* **9**: 174–186.

Lewis LK, Maher C, Belanger K, Tremblay M, Chaput JP, Olds T (2016) At the mercy of the gods: associations between weather, physical activity and sedentary time in children. *Pediatric Exercise Science* **28**: 152–163.

Longmuir P, Bar-Or O (2000) Factors influencing the physical activity levels of youths with physical and sensory disabilities. *Adapted Physical Activity Quarterly* **17**: 40–53.

Maher C (2008) *Using the Internet to Increase Physical Activity in Adolescents with Cerebral Palsy – Are You Kidding?* Doctoral dissertation, School of Health Sciences, University of South Australia.

Maher C, Kenyon A, McEvoy M, Sprod J (2013) The reliability and validity of a research-grade pedometer for children and adolescents with cerebral palsy. *Developmental Medicine and Child Neurology* 55: 827–833.

Maher C, Williams M, Olds T, Lane A (2007) Physical and sedentary activity in adolescents with cerebral palsy. *Developmental Medicine and Child Neurology* 49: 450–457.

McIver K, Brown W, Pfeiffer K, Dowda M, Pate R (2016) Development and testing of the observational system for recording physical activity in children: elementary school. *Res Q Exerc Sport* 87: 101–109.

Nooijen C, De Groot J, Stam H, Van den Berg-Emons R, Bussmann H (2015) Validation of an activity monitor for children who are partly or completely wheelchair-dependent. *Journal of Neuroengineering and Rehabilitation* 12: 11.

Olds T, Ridley K, Dollman J, Maher C (2010) The validity of a computerized use of time recall, the Multimedia Activity Recall for Children and adolescents. *Pediatric Exercise Science* 22: 34.

Park J, Kazuko I, Kim E, Kim J, Yoon J (2014) Estimating free-living human energy expenditure: practical aspects of the doubly labeled water method and its applications. *Nutr Res Pract* 8: 241–248.

Psota T, Chen K (2013) Measuring energy expenditure in clinical populations: rewards and challenges. *Eur J Clin Nutr* 67: 446–442.

Ridley K (2005) *The Multimedia Activity Recall for Children and Adolescents (MARCA): Development and Validation.* PhD thesis, School of Health Sciences, University of South Australia.

Rodriguez G, Beghin L, Michaud L, Moreno L, Turck D, Gottrand F (2002) Comparison of the TriTrac-R3D accelerometer and a self-report activity diary with heart-rate monitoring for the assessment of energy expenditure in children. *British Journal of Nutrition* 87: 623–631.

Rowe P, Schuldheisz J, Van der Mars H (1997) Validation of SOFIT for measuring physical activity of first- to eighth-grade students. *Pediatric Exercise Science* 9: 136–149.

Sala DA, Grissom HE, Delsole EM et al. (2019) Measuring ambulation with wrist-based and hip-based activity trackers for children with cerebral palsy. *Developmental Medicine & Child Neurology* 61: 1309–1313.

Silcott N, Bassett DJ, Thompson D, Fitzhugh E, Steeves J (2011) Evaluation of the Omron HJ-720ITC pedometer under free-living conditions. *Medicine and Science in Sports and Exercise* 43: 1791–1797.

Sirard J, Pate R (2001) Physical activity assessment in children and adolescents. *Sports Medicine* 31: 439–454.

Takken T, Van der Net J, Kuis W, Helders, P (2003) Physical activity and health related physical fitness in children with juvenile idiopathic arthritis. *Ann Rheum Dis* 62: 885–889.

Telford A, Salmon J, Jolley D, Crawford D (2004) Reliability and validity of physical activity questionnaires for children: the Children's Leisure Activities Study Survey (CLASS). *Pediatric Exercise Science* 16: 64–78.

Trost S (2005) Discussion paper for the development of recommendations for children's and youths' participation in health promoting physical activity. *Australian Department of Health and Ageing.* Canberra ACT: Australian Government.

Trost S (2007) State of the art reviews: measurement of physical activity in children and adolescents. *American Journal of Lifestyle Medicine* 1: 299–314.

Trost S, Morgan A, Saunders R, Felton G, Ward D, Pate R (2000). Children's understanding of the concept of physical activity. *Pediatric Exercise Science* **12**: 293–299.

Trost S, O'Neill M (2013) Clinical use of objective measures of physical activity. *Br J Sports Med* **48**: 178–181.

Tudor Locke C, Barreira T, Schuna JJ et al. (2015) Improving wear time compliance with a 24-hour waist-worn accelerometer protocol in the International Study of Childhood Obesity, Lifestyle and the Environment (ISCOLE). *Int J Behav Nutr Phys Act* **12**: 11.

Warren J, Ekelund U, Besson H et al. (2010) Assessment of physical activity – a review of methodologies with reference to epidemiological research: a report of the exercise physiology section of the European Association of Cardiovascular Prevention and Rehabilitation. *European Journal of Preventive Cardiology* **17**: 127–139.

White L, Volfson Z, Faulkner G, Arbour-Nicitopoulos K (2016) Reliability and validity of physical activity instruments used in children and youth with physical disabilities: a systematic review. *Pediatric Exercise Science* **28**: 240–263.

Young N, Williams J, Yoshida K, Wright J (2000) Measurement properties of the Activities Scale for Kids. *J Clin Epidemiol* **53**: 125–137.

CHAPTER 5

How to Promote a Physically Active Lifestyle Across the Lifespan

Ine Wigernaes, Berit Gjessing, Anne Ottestad, and Kjersti Syvertsen

PRINCIPLES OF BEHAVIOUR CHANGE

Overview

Numerous theories address behavioural change and the elements within – the desire to change into something more attractive including the ambiguity between pros and cons. Consciousness of one's own habits and status at the moment is one element. Consider, in addition, the experiences that have provided energy and self-efficacy, and belief in one's own power to change. All of these may be summarized as 'motivation to change'.

Actions and initiatives are opposite to passivism and conservatism. At first glance, motivation may overlap with optimism. Lack of motivation may be similar to discouragement. Is motivation contagious from one life area to another? Will a person who loses interest in education or learning also be unmotivated in other areas in life, possibly leading to loneliness, physical deterioration, and depression?

Human beings can be proactive and engaged or, alternatively, passive and alienated, largely as impacted by the social conditions in which they develop and function. Many factors are examined that enhance versus undermine intrinsic motivation, self-regulation, and well-being.

The simplicity of motivation in making small and large choices is both a beauty and a threat. Daniel Kahneman wisely postulated the brain's need to make a plan, reduce the degrees of freedom, and create structure in order to establish persistent habits (Kahneman 2011). This also holds in critical phases and grave and desperate life situations. The beauty lies in the process, which demands few or no external aids; the threat describes our disbelief in the everyday rhythm, the repetitions, and simplicity itself and the 'power of Tuesdays'.

One of the most powerful indicators of health is belief in the future (World Health Organization 1999). The conviction that an individual has the power to improve a certain situation is called empowerment, which is also described as the strength to actually make efforts in a desired direction. Being aware of one's own resources and regularly reminding ourselves about, and seeking experiences at, an adapted level, is regarded as substantial.

Theories and models of human behaviour have been derived from all disciplines of the social sciences. The various theories of how lifestyle is generated or changed are more complementary than conflicting, and focus on both the individual and environmental aspects of people's lives. The use of theories of behaviour holds for lifestyle, consumption, environmental sustainability, and responsibility (Jackson 2005).

In the famous dialogue *Meno*, Plato and Socrates argued that 'He who knows what good is will do good' (IvyPanda 2021). This provides a rather insufficient description of promoting behaviours. Therefore, Knowledge, Attitude, Practice remains just a theory. The multifactorial benefits of changing an inactive lifestyle into some physical activity are well known, and new international guidelines on physical activity and sedentary behaviour were recently launched by the World Health Organization (2020). Still, only 30% of the adult population in Norway fulfils the advice from national health authorities of 30 minutes of light physical activity daily (FHI 2022). Children are advised to be active for 1 hour every day. Six-year-olds mostly fulfil this, but activity levels are reduced to 50% and below at 15 years. However, assessing activity constitutes challenges regarding definition, self-report, and inadequate understanding of intensity and activity (FHI 2022) (see Chapter 4).

Theories of Behavioural Change

Individually focused theories of behaviour (change) are often criticized. Few, if any, individuals are considered isolated from the rest of the world. However, individual models of behaviour are strongly intuitive, evident, and explicit, especially when considered against the complex and diffuse impacts of social structures. The following theories of behaviour change are described in this chapter:

1. Stages of Change Model (Prochaska 1979)
2. Social Cognitive Theory (Bandura 1986)

3. Sense of Coherence Theory (Antonovsky 1996)
4. Self-determination Theory (Ryan and Deci 2000)
5. Theory of Planned Behaviour (Ajzen 1991)
6. Social Practice Theory (Chatterton 2011)
7. 4Es Model (Jackson 2005)
8. MINDSPACE Framework (Dolan et al. 2010).

(1) The **Stages of Change Model** (Prochaska 1979) is widely used in counselling and motivational interviewing for lifestyle change in young people and adults. Its use with small children has to our knowledge not been described. It uses (i) pre-contemplation, (ii) contemplation, (iii) preparation, (iv) action, and (v) maintenance as imaginary steps towards a change, making the individuals identify the pros and cons of changing behaviour, thereby proposing solutions and concrete actions themselves.

(2) Invaluable aspects of individual, social, and societal perspectives are included in the **Social Cognitive Theory** (Bandura 1986). The theoretical components are: **modelling, outcome expectancies, self-efficacy, and identification**. Modelling and defaulting what is tolerable and common in smaller or larger societies will play a role. Furthermore, what is meaningful for the individual and whether it actually works, in terms of being effective, will influence adherence to new habits. Sex, age, and cultural context will be crucial factors for what is meaningful to an individual person. Children will have totally different interests than adults.

Self-efficacy is 'the belief in one's capabilities to organize and execute the courses of action required to manage prospective situations' (Bandura 1986). This core belief affects each of the basic processes of personal change. From an early age, individual self-efficacy plays a major role in how goals, tasks, and challenges are approached and developed. Individuals who have developed high self-efficacy from early childhood are more likely to believe they can master challenging problems and recover more quickly from setbacks and disappointments (Bandura 1986). Individuals with low self-efficacy are characterized by lack of self-confidence, low expectations of one's own performance, and avoiding challenging tasks. Therefore, self-efficacy plays a central role in behaviour performance, including various health-related situations such as weight loss and quitting smoking. Self-efficacy has produced some of the most consistent results associated with an increase in participation in exercise (FHI 2022).

All individuals have experiences from early childhood. Earlier defeats or embarrassments, exclusion, and ridicule, are placed on the negative side of the mathematical equation of motivation. Thus, creating new experiences and constantly reminding oneself about good feelings and mastery makes the negative experiences vague, blurry, and less significant (Bandura 1986).

(3) According to Aaron Antonovsky's **Sense of Coherence Theory**, a sense of coherence develops from early childhood and consists of three components: **manageability, meaningfulness, and comprehensibility** (Antonovsky 1996). *Manageability* develops from early experiences of coping and mastery. When a child regularly and sufficiently experiences that the challenges in daily life are manageable with the available resources, a sense of manageability develops. *Meaningfulness* develops from early experiences of goal attainment. When a child sufficiently often reaches self-determined goals with available resources in daily life, a sense of meaningfulness develops, as the child learns that struggling is worthwhile. *Comprehensibility* develops from early experience of predictability. When a child regularly and sufficiently experiences having control over activities and events in everyday life with the available resources, a sense of comprehensibility develops (Antonovsky 1996). In sum, these experiences serve as 'general resistance resources', which develop early and are relatively stable through life. Thus, they can be useful when meeting challenges in daily life (Antonovsky 1996).

(4) In the **Self-determination Theory**, Deci and Ryan postulate three innate psychological needs: **competence, autonomy, and relatedness**. *Competence,* as in control and mastery and a felt sense of confidence in a social context, is not a skill or capability attained in an objective sense but is strongly related to self-efficacy, which is developed from early experiences (Ryan and Deci 2000).

Autonomy is related to initiatives and the feeling of representing one's own choices. Therefore, children should be asked about their preferences for different physical activities. This implies choosing physical activity regardless of rewards, enforcement, or punishment. The feeling of being an 'agent for your own actions' connects to an identity as 'being an active person', and contributes to the choices made. This identity is also a strong predictor of staying physically active as an adult (Ryan and Deci 2000; FHI 2022).

Relatedness implies a real bonding to others and the feeling of being a participant (Ryan and Deci 2000). Relatedness is one of the core elements in the recently developed model and framework of participation for persons with disabilities (Imms et al. 2017). The stories of the *Upturn* group and the *Beito-gang* (lived experiences later in this chapter), illustrate how the sense of belonging develops when being in a context where there are others with similar challenges. Both children and adults with disabilities sometimes need such 'safe contexts' to form experiences that nurture internalization of the sense of belonging (Imms et al. 2017). To meet 'someone like me' is also important in relation to perhaps having another role, not always being the only one who needs help or the last person to cross the line. Interventions need to create situations and processes where actors are free to reflect critically on their actions and the context in which they act. The relatedness and autonomy underlines this point (Ryan and Deci 2000).

(5) *Intention to act* has repeatedly predicted behaviour. Intention is itself a summary of the combination of attitudes towards a behaviour. This includes the evaluation of the positive or negative expected outcomes, the social pressures and perceptions of what others think they should do, and their likelihood to comply with these. A close parallel to self-efficacy was added in the **Theory of Planned Behaviour**, as a third set of factors that affects intention (and behaviour). Perceived behavioural control is a belief of level of difficulty with which the individual may perform the behaviour (Ajzen 1991). Evidence suggests that the planned behaviour can predict 20% to 30% of the variance in behaviour resulting from interventions and even a greater proportion of intention. Both the attitudes towards the behaviour and perceived behavioural control components of the theory show strong correlations to behaviour itself. To date, only weak correlations have been established between behaviour and subjective norms (Ajzen and Adden 1986). However, using the theory to explain and predict likely behaviour may be a useful method for identifying particular influences on behaviour that could be targeted for change (Munro et al. 2007).

(6) **Social Practice Theory** is something of an umbrella approach under which various aspects of theory are pursued (Chatterton 2011). This theory addresses three elements: **materials, meanings, and procedures**. The *materials* are the physical objects that permit or facilitate certain activities to be performed in specific ways (sports equipment or transportation are good examples). The *meanings* are images, interpretations, or concepts associated with activities that determine how and when they might be performed. Education as a preparation for the preferred skill level, and creation of an inner picture of yourself in the activity, are important in order to develop an identity. The *procedures* are skills, knowledge, or competencies that permit or lead to activities being undertaken in certain ways. Learning the hard way and improving after struggling might be such procedures (Chatterton 2011). This holds for both children and adults. Experiences of making a change most often create pride and a possible transfer to other life arenas. An anxious person who manages to meet neighbours or classmates for a walk or to go to a café once a week will most probably feel general empowerment, activity competence, a new sense of self, and, eventually, a change of identity. 'I managed this, which I would have never thought 1 year ago, so now I might join the "gym group" as well.'

Our biology and body represent potentials, like more favourable characteristics, such as a robust immune system. Similarly, accumulating knowledge indicates that most physical traits are trainable, like speed, strength, endurance, coordination, and flexibility. In addition, learning from or imitating family members, friends, and colleagues may widen our perspectives on what is possible. This is of great importance when it comes to creating habits and building physical and mental strength. A child that observes a father who manages to quit smoking, or a mother who creates space and empowers herself to engage in some physical activity once a week, is learning that it is possible to change habits and promote better ones.

(7) The **4Es Model** is also applied in politics (Jackson 2005) and advocates behaviour change strategies under four categories: **enable, encourage, engage, and exemplify**. Additionally, the model states that in more examples where behaviour is entrenched or habitual, the government uses catalysts to enhance people to behave differently, like raising the price on cigarettes, sugar, and liquor, lowering the prices on vegetables, and an overall area plan that includes conservation of green areas and walking paths. All of these actions reflect values. Behaviours and attitudes of individual consumers are at the core of this model and the majority of interventions (information, education, incentives) are aimed at affecting individual choices.

(8) The **MINDSPACE Framework** is described by simple keywords that further describe central elements (Dolan et al. 2010). **Messenger:** Both children and adults are heavily influenced by who communicates information. A friend, a parent, a professional, a celebrity, someone we trust or dislike for any of many reasons will influence our choices. **Incentives:** Our responses to incentives are shaped by predictable mental shortcuts, such as strongly avoiding losses. What are my chances? What is in this for me? Does it work for someone like me, or my child? **Norms:** We are strongly influenced by what others of the same age, sex, and social class do. **Defaults:** We 'go with the flow' of pre-set options. Close relatives and relations are hiding or uncovering possibilities. Copying local actions may aid in ignoring or creating obstacles. **Salience:** Both children's and adults' attention is drawn to what is novel and seems relevant to us. What is new and interesting information that suits my identity and image? **Priming:** Our acts are often influenced by subconscious cues, brought along from early experiences during childhood or information that is processed and acted upon. **Affect:** Our emotional associations can powerfully shape our actions, as described in the 'engage' part of the 4Es Model. The experience of feeling calm and happy after shovelling snow, learning that an initial assumption of 'work – tired – boring', may in fact lead to 'meaningful – strong – fun'. **Commitments:** We seek to be consistent with our public promises and reciprocate acts. **Ego:** Both children and adults act in ways that make us feel better about ourselves. This brings along the need for creating our own experiences that will outline the theories and keywords.

Strategies for Overcoming Barriers to Being Physically Active

Studies on motivation and participation bring to the fore the larger perspectives of research on a population with physical disabilities and are often described as a magnifier of general findings. The variation within this group will most likely be just as large as in any other population. However, in recent large studies, both children and adults with chronic disabilities have been shown to be less physically active than their non-disabled peers (Saebu 2011). A belief has been established in rehabilitation services that high motivation for physical activity is caused by health benefits for this population. Furthermore, an assumption of reduced physical health and poor accessibility to activity and activity aids has been a basis of knowledge (Saebu and Sorensen 2011). Access to facilities, recreational parks, forests, tracks and trails, weight rooms, gyms, aerobic or yoga classes, team sports, or creating possibility to cycle/walk to school or the workplace is often a political issue (Saebu and Sorensen 2011). If apples are offered at every corner, most people would eat apples; the same holds for offering a pint of beer. Accessibility will make the cognitive decision-making process shorter and promote autonomy. The same idea holds for preparation for participation: putting out food, clothes, and equipment, and making arrangement of transportation.

However, Saebu and Sorensen (2011) showed that individual factors like intrinsic motivation and identity have far more influence than previously believed, and suggest the need for more interventions aimed at strengthening the individual factors from an early age, in addition to the physical and social environmental factors. Having fun, being with friends and 'owning' responsibility for the initiative are of far greater importance than a doctor who tells you to exercise, or establishing and nourishing bad conscience for not eating enough carrots. Degree of disability and rewards were also of less importance than presumed (Saebu et al. 2013).

Motivated persons are proud to overcome barriers, while the others may blame the barrier itself. If finances are a barrier, seek second-hand equipment on the internet or set up a list of activities that demand fewer investments. Inner motivation may be strengthened within a rehabilitation programme where the autonomy and experience and being agent for one's own priorities and choices are emphasized in addition to social support by being part of a group (Saebu et al. 2013). Parents, peers, coaches, and health care professionals may play an extrinsic role as primers and facilitators for a focus on benefits. The individual question could be phrased: 'Who would (I like to) support me in this process?'

It is well known that high socioeconomic status is a reliable predictor for choosing an active lifestyle. One should be careful drawing direct conclusions about causality. Whether it is the academic performance or wealth itself, or more probably an indirect consequence of more flexible working hours, as opposed to scheduled/blue-collar-labour that gives excess energy, is unknown (World Health Organization 2020).

Being aware of the power of good feelings in order to remain motivated and achieve goals is called the golden window of opportunity. Identification of these may be a prerequisite for change instead of being in the 'Monday, I'll initiate another strict diet programme' lane. Windows of opportunity give a boost of energy and self-confidence that may fuel and propel a desired change. The right moment might be after a vacation or rehabilitation programme.

> **At Every Intersection: You Have a Choice**
>
> Well known in Norway, Kristian Fjellanger has developed a talk-show about 'my life as a fat-so'. Weighing 183kg at age 30 years, he figured that something needed to be done. Interestingly, on his way 'up' to 183kg, decisions regarding eating and inactivity behaviour had been taken for more than a decade, probably unconsciously and automatically. Being aware that every time he decides to eat or sit down he is at an intersection, which may be a first step towards empowerment – being in charge of own decisions – and motivation for change, means that each time he may choose differently.
>
> He started reading and started to prepare. He learned that creating a new habit would take 60 days. He expected the first 60 days to be painful. He had a 4-week vacation due to working additional hours, and claimed this point to be crucial: 'In order to manage the change I needed energy.'

In the 1990s the Hungarian psychologist, Mihyaly Csíkszentmihályi, often mentioned as the most prominent researcher within the field of positive psychology, created the idea of 'flow' as a situation where a person was fully in accordance with abilities and challenges (Csíkszentmihályi 1998). Matching the relation (ability–challenge) is a pre-requisite, and underlines the adaptation of the activity for children or adults with or without disabilities. Although the terminology has been used for high performance situations, flow is used on a daily basis by everyone. Finding that optimal level for each individual will never go out of style. However, it is increasingly difficult to set internal goals when research, health authorities, and commercial forces constantly communicate efficient training programmes, optimal weight loss, and 'what is best for you'. This poses the following important question: 'what is possible, desirable, and achievable for me – now – with my resources?'

Basic Steps for Initiating Behavioural Change Towards a More Active Lifestyle

An analysis of one's own life situation will most often be a necessary initial step to identify network, resources, time, facilities, and one's own preferences and goals.

- What are my own, or my child's, old negative experiences to be dealt with?
- When do I, or my child, feel successful? What are my, or my child's, resources?
  - Continue and complete the following sentence: 'I am good at …'
- Who can help me by giving advice, holding my hand, making appointments, making me strong?
- Is it possible for me to go for a short walk? Can I do floor exercises indoors while watching the news? Only 20 minutes would break the normal routine and establish new ones.
- What are my short-term goals for myself and my child?

Getting to know yourself and your family's habits will create routines that are easy to adhere to. Some of the most successful weight-reduction programmes start with this writing-down-awareness-strategy. This needs to be followed by a simple set of routines that includes: sit down when eating, eat slowly, write down what you eat and ask yourself: Why do I, or my child, need to eat more now? Do we need more food?

Recognition of the power of everyday habits must be underlined. Books, shows, speeches, articles about 'I lost 100kg', 'I climbed Kilimanjaro without legs', or 'I cross-country skied across the South Pole being blind' may be of some importance, but focus instead on an awareness of one's own habits, schedules, barriers, and mastering arenas. Being aware of motivational 'risk periods' is necessary, such as a restart after a flu or an injury, or storing sweets and crisps in the house if you wish to eat more healthily. According to Kahneman's philosophy, eating a banana or a sandwich in advance prevents both children and adults from cravings while passing the shelves of chocolate in the grocery store. However, it requires planning and the banana needs to be right there (Kahneman 2011).

Campaigns seem to have limited effects, although some are better than others: 'I am not fast, but I am 100% sure that I am better than the ones staying on the couch.' Avoiding bad breath and having kissable lips are probably more graspable and short-term goals for a teenager when it comes to quitting smoking than lecturing on the statistical risk for obtaining lung cancer at age 76 years (Kahneman 2011).

> In rehabilitation at Beitostølen Healthsports Center, the invaluable element of 'free space – closed place' is specifically mentioned by all users with a large variation in disabilities or their parents, from preschool children to elderly people. The repetitive practice: you fall, hurt yourself, look silly – and try again intensively, and eventually succeed, all the while with peers with different disabilities around. Pedagogues and health professionals are present. Getting used to clothing, food, adjustments, what to bring 'in case of ...' creates lots of learning and experiences. This seeks to promote lower thresholds, autonomy, and self-efficacy, which are transferrable geographically and to other life arenas (Willis et al. 2018).

USING ASSISTIVE DEVICES AND OTHER TECHNOLOGY TO DO PHYSICAL ACTIVITY

For many people with disabilities, a well-adjusted assistive device is essential for their opportunity to participate in an activity regardless of age. Studies show that lack of suitable equipment is one of several reasons for low activity levels both in children and adults (Engel-Yeger et al. 2009; Bedell et al. 2013). Assistive devices for leisure activities are equipment that is specifically designed to help individuals with disabilities to participate in play and sports (Gjessing et al. 2018). Examples are an arm-propelled cycle, a bicycle with an assistive motor, a motorized chair for floor ball, and a sit-ski and balance-frame for cross-country skiing. Many individuals with childhood-onset physical disabilities need adaptation of activities in order to participate satisfactorily.

The availability of assistive devices differs from country to country. Several countries have systems for public funding of such devices, seeking to give equal opportunities of assistive devices regardless of socioeconomic status.

Principles for Device Selection

When acquiring an assistive device (i.e. if a wheelchair user wants an arm-cycle for participation reasons), selection of an appropriate bicycle and proper adaptation of this bicycle are essential (Gjessing et al. 2018). Individuals have different needs based on demographics, geography, activity preference, and individual capacity. A number of arm-cycle alternatives exist. Cooperation between a professional and the user is essential in order to find the most suitable equipment. The professional is often a physiotherapist or occupational therapist. Local variation in competence regarding assistive devices is significant. Educating professionals in order to enhance knowledge of selecting and adapting assistive devices has to be emphasized. Giving more people with physical disabilities the opportunity to participate in physical activities and the selection of the best equipment to support this is vital.

A study on the experiences of children and young people with acquiring and using assistive devices showed the variation when trying new equipment (Gjessing et al. 2018). Some expressed that it is obvious how to use the equipment and initiate the activity immediately, while others were sceptical about trying out new equipment. 'How fast will I go? Will I manage it? What if I don't? Can anyone see me?' are among their explicit concerns. In such situations, presence of a confident and experienced professional or a peer role model can be very helpful. A role model is often an older person with a comparable disability or situation, who may manage the same assistive device.

> Jacob is about to learn sit-ski with his father in the alpine area. An instructor on alpine skis is telling him how to do it, but Jacob does not quite manage. He is starting to be a bit frustrated when another man in a sit-ski comes towards him and says 'hi!' Jacob recognizes the fellow from the day before and knows that he uses a wheelchair, just like himself. The man willingly offers to show Jacob how to ski. Jacob observes with great enjoyment, especially how he uses his crutch skis when performing downhill turns. Jacob thinks that the task is difficult, but now he is determined to make it!

Self-efficacy is a product of experiences, skill, feedback, persuasion, and intentions. Therefore, individuals with low self-efficacy benefit from additional time in a safe environment, with professionals and preferably also role models (Bandura 1986; Willis et al. 2018). After mastering a task and getting confident, it is desirable to return to peers in the local environment and in real-life settings. Many children and adults with disabilities highlight the importance of activity devices that make them more independent while being active. Dependency on assistance with operating the assistive device, on the other hand, is reported to be a barrier for using the equipment (Gjessing et al. 2018).

In rehabilitation programmes for persons with physical disabilities, interventions are often based on principles of adapting the contextual factors (Darrah et al. 2011; Palisano et al. 2012; Rosenbaum and Gorter 2012). Darrah et al. (2011) describe 'context therapy' as a suitable approach. The focus is increasingly put on identifying each person's abilities, and on establishing procedures and treatments based on these abilities. The method is characterized not by changing the person's impairments but rather on facilitating the task and/or adapting the environment, so that the task can be implemented with success. This method has similarities with adapted physical activity, where the purpose is to adapt activities to the person's conditions (Sherrill 2004). Real-life experiences facilitate development of skills that optimize participation. Such competencies could be social, physical, or technical.

Assistive Devices in Activity: Bridging the Social Gap?

The importance of the environment for participation in physical activity is highlighted in an increasing number of scientific articles (Heah et al. 2007; Darrah et al. 2011; Palisano et al. 2012, Rosenbaum and Gorter 2012). One of the most important factors that motivate children and young people to use their assistive devices in leisure activities is being with friends and sharing experiences with them (Gjessing et al. 2018). Obviously, children depend on their family in the first years of their lives (Rosenbaum and Gorter 2012). The family is also the most important facilitator for both social interactions and activity for this population. When children turn 9 to 10 years old, it becomes increasingly important to join peers and 'significant others' at the expense of close family (Allender et al. 2006; Anaby et al. 2013; Nyquist et al. 2016). Several children with childhood-onset physical disabilities experience not being able to keep up with peers in activities (Heah et al. 2007). As they grow older, comparison with peers will most likely progress, which may lead to more isolation. Both children and adults with disabilities participate less frequently and have less environmental support in the community, compared to persons without disabilities (Darrah et al. 2011; Sebire et al. 2013). Simultaneously, it is agreed that support from peers promotes participation (Blair and Morris 2009; Sebire et al. 2013). Children with disabilities, who are less physically active with friends, lose the advantage of peer support in joint activities, and hence participate less in environments where friendships and an identity as physically active are developed. However, those who do participate with friends have better opportunities for peer support that might lead to even more and continuous participation. Relatedness and real bonding to others are prerequisites for sustained behaviour (Ryan and Deci 2000).

Assistive Devices and Intrinsic Motivation: Sliding Doors

Even though lack of equipment and facilities to perform activities are barriers for participation in physical activities, as said above, Saebu and Sorensen (2011) found that intrinsic motivation and development of an identity as a physically active person might be the most important factors for choosing to participate in physical activity as adults.

This is supported by Sebire et al. (2013), who found intrinsic motivation to be the only type of motivation that can be associated with children's physical activity levels. Since it is important to maintain physical activity from childhood into adulthood (Ryan and Deci 2000), it is beneficial to identify and encourage activity behaviours that are driven by intrinsic motivation. However, children who use adapted equipment in physical activity express that intrinsic motivation is just one of several factors that are important for being able to perform the activity (Darrah et al. 2011). Environmental factors like adaptation of the equipment and peer support seem equally important for maintaining physical activity into adulthood (Sebire et al. 2013). These two factors will potentially mutually enhance each other. Assistive devices and adapted equipment may play a key role in creating the window of opportunity to experience intrinsic motivation and the ability to participate with peers. These factors should therefore be examined carefully for each individual, regardless of age.

UPTURN: A PRACTICAL EXAMPLE OF A TRAINING GROUP FOR CHILDREN AND YOUNG PEOPLE WITH DISABILITIES

Cooperation Between Community Sports Clubs and Physiotherapists in a Local Municipality

Twenty years ago, adapted leisure activities for children with physical disabilities, in Bærum Municipality outside Oslo, were extremely limited. Some individual follow-up by physiotherapists during school hours was available. However, the ever-increasing budget constraints led to insufficient funding of organized exercise groups at the relevant schools. A physiotherapist and a rehabilitation coordinator in the municipality initiated a collaborative project with a community sports club, aiming at providing adapted recreational activities with the opportunity to create an active social community. They contacted Beitostølen Healthsports Centre (BHC) to book a stay for a group of children and young people with disabilities from Bærum. This fitted in well with the BHC project, which was called 'the local environment model'.

Next, the local initiators and the municipality invited a group of children and young people to weekly training sessions in order to motivate them to apply for a group stay at BHC and to become a confident and tight-knit group prior to the stay. The municipality did an excellent job during several information meetings in the period ahead of the application deadline. All the children who participated in the activity group applied for the stay.

The publicly funded stay at BHC was a fantastic experience for the children and parents involved. The parents were also given sufficient time to become acquainted with each other and to discuss how to continue the activity group. It was clearly communicated that in the long-term the group could no longer continue under the auspices of the municipality. Therefore, it was necessary that a sports team was established based on voluntary efforts. Fossum Sports Association welcomed the group, and three parents took responsibility for managing the activities in the group. *Upturn* was established as part of Fossum Sports Association in 2004.

Upturn

Upturn was marketed as an adapted all-sports group for children with physical impairments from 7 to 17 years. The programme consisted of one exercise session per week, and the activities on offer rotated between sports-hall-based and outdoor activities. The activities were varied and play-centred, with a focus on accomplishment, social interaction, and cooperation. One of the goals was that the participants should be able to try out many different activities. Besides the typical sports-hall activities, others included climbing, rowing, skating sessions, bowling, curling, golf, swimming, archery, tae kwon do, and fishing trips.

The underlying idea was that *Upturn* should be a door opener into regular groups in Fossum Sports Association, with football, orienteering, as well as cross-country and alpine skiing. However, it soon became clear that the atmosphere in the group became so strong and tightly knit that everyone in the group preferred to continue training within the safe parameters created by *Upturn*. Although the other groups in Fossum Sports Association were extremely positive and inclusive, it was the *Upturn* group that 'kept to themselves'. Cooperation with other groups in Fossum Sports Association resulted in events, such as biathlon and star orienteering, as well as adapted cross-country skiing and slalom training during the course of 4 weeks every winter.

Upturn worked as a platform that generated further activity groups and small networks. Some of those involved started climbing, horseback riding, swimming, or training together at fitness centres. Several also became good friends and spent a great deal of spare time together.

The young people, who 'grew out of' *Upturn* were offered the opportunity to continue their training in another local sports club, Friskis & Svettis, which means Fit & Sweaty. There, around 15 young people with disabilities meet once a week for strength training with qualified guidance by instructors and assistant coaches. One assistant coach has cerebral palsy himself and was previously part of *Upturn*. Like *Upturn*, this is a low-threshold activity with focus on social interaction, safe boundaries, enthusiasm for exercise, and accomplishment of training goals. Even though the programme is facilitated, all activities take place at the same time as the other activities in the sports club.

What Did *Upturn* Mean for the Participants?

It is easy for young people with disabilities to become excluded at school because they are unable to keep up physically. They often cannot take part in the social settings formed by groups walking to and from school, nor are they able to join in the same leisure activities. Social networks fail them. *Upturn* is an extremely important social arena for the children and young people involved. Many have made friends with whom they still spend a great deal of time.

The good team spirit in the group meant they dared to take on more challenges. They were motivated to try new things without fear of embarrassing themselves. For participants in the *Upturn* group, many exciting activities were offered in addition to more ordinary sports-hall activities. This is what their typically developing peers experienced during physical education classes, while those with disabilities previously sat on the side line or experienced painful defeats. The experiences from *Upturn* served as discussion points at school; they conferred status among their fellow students.

There was a focus on mastery experiences in *Upturn*. However, the coach was extremely confident in his role and was able to motivate, challenge, and be considerate. There was structure and order to the training sessions. The children had to relate to each other and adhere to rules – they were simply treated like any other children. In *Upturn*, it was possible to compete – play as a team and bring out the best in each other. During physical education at school, many felt that they were the reason for the team's defeat. For the first time, many gained the experience of 'achieving' at a higher level than others, and they could, with great satisfaction, lend a helping hand to those who needed and wanted it. The adapted training made it possible to 'exert oneself' in the right way and gain a feeling of mastery in doing a little better than the time before.

How was it Operated?

Two main factors contributed to the success of *Upturn*: the close cooperation between the municipality and the reliable coaches with a high level of expertise in the field of adaptation.

The municipality provided economic support by employing two assistant coaches, and the municipality's physiotherapists actively recruited new children into the group. At the same time, they contributed their expertise as professionals when necessary. The physiotherapists' active participation provided reassurance for parents unsure whether sports were appropriate for their children.

The municipality was also an active promoter of visits by *Upturn* to BHC. These stays were inspirational and improved cohesion among the children as well as among the parents, creating a sense of belonging and experiences of new social roles, and learning new skills that could be continued at home. The freedom of choice regarding activities, increased activity competence, and sense of self along with good team spirit were important factors behind the *Upturn* group's participation in a series of sporting events and social trips (Ryan and Deci 2000; Imms et al. 2017).

Ever since its inception, there has been a focus in *Upturn* on employing young, cool coaches with robust expertise in adaptation, as well as on reinforcing the coaching team with assistants in order for parents to avoid participating and assisting during training. Thanks to financial support from the municipality, the coaches received competitive wages for their work, and they were reliable and brilliant role models. They were creative with organizing activities and were confident in their role of both providing challenges and being considerate. The role of the parents consisted largely of administering the group and applying for funds, as well as marketing the programme in cooperation with the municipality.

CHALLENGING FACTORS

The activities on offer in *Upturn* were adapted for children and young people with primarily physical impairments. An ever-growing proportion of participants with significant cognitive challenges made it difficult to create a satisfactory training programme for everyone. The composition of the group became unclear, and parents of children with motor challenges hesitated to send their children to exercise with peers with intellectual disability.

The original core group of children and parents left *Upturn* as the children grew out of the programme. Filling the vacant positions with new recruits was not successful, neither with children nor with enthusiastic parents. *Upturn* no longer falls under the specific tasks of the physiotherapist in Bærum municipality.

The experiences gained from *Upturn* demonstrate the importance of providing an adapted training programme embedded in an established sports club, which is able to assist with any necessary administrative help, showing that both individual and environmental factors and structures are important for sustained adapted physical activity (Saebu and Sorensen 2011). At its peak, there were almost 35 children and young people in *Upturn*, which continued for 15 years.

THE *BEITO-GANG*

In 1996 a group of 14 adults with different disabilities from the same local municipality, Hurum, were at a rehabilitation stay at BHC (www.bhss.no/aktuelt/). During this stay, the group members developed friendships, common engagement, and importantly, confidence that their experiences had to be shared with others in similar life situations. After 4 weeks at BHC more than 20 years ago, the group returned home with a lot of inspiration and started to train together once a week with local professionals. The *Beito-gang*, which they called themselves, had initiated a popular training group, and more people joined the training sessions. This openness to new members was an important factor for the sustainability of the group.

After a while, the group got financial support from the county administration and was formalized as Hurum Healthsports Club. Since then, 550 persons have been members of this healthsports club, and in 2016, the club had 300 paying members. The club organizes weekly training in a sports hall, outdoor walks, as well as sessions in a swimming pool. In addition, they arrange six excursions yearly, sometimes to BHC for a 'first love revival'. Through all these years, a small enthusiastic team has hosted this club.

The enthusiastic team behind this initiative is proud of having been able to accomplish this dream. There is no doubt that this is a good example of collaboration between a rehabilitation institution in the specialist health care system, local health professionals, and voluntary enthusiasts in the local community. The competence of the professionals at BHC with adapted physical activity influenced the group from Hurum in 1996. What these group members learned they brought back to their local community, where adults with different special needs can still enjoy training together in everyday life. Again, participation in preferred activities, experiences of increased activity competence, and sense of self and social belonging, contributed to sustained physical activity (Ryan and Deci 2000; Imms et al. 2017).

CONCLUDING REMARKS

Asking older people who succeed in keeping a social network, appreciating life, embracing events, even if the physical limits are obvious to a younger population, would probably add to existing knowledge in the area.

In between academic theories and political facilitation, one should consider the Nike Inc. slogan 'Just Do It.' Attention should focus on the need to create experiences repeatedly. Bear in mind that the first 10 times, and the first 60 days may be painful, boring, and include additional hassle and minimal feelings of mastery. This is the reality for achieving physical activity goals and is how autonomous adherence to healthy behaviour should be communicated.

REFERENCES

Ajzen IM (1991) The theory of planned behaviour. *Organisational Behaviour and Human Decision Processes* **50**: 179–211. 10.1016/0749-5978(91)90020-T.

Ajzen I, Madden TJ (1986) Prediction of goal directed behavior: attitudes, intentions, and perceived behavioral control. *Journal of Experimental Social Psychology* **22**: 453–474.

Allender S, Cowburn G, Foster C (2006) Understanding participation in sport and physical activity among children and adults: a review of qualitative studies. *Health Education Research* **21**: 826–835. 10.1093/her/cyl063.

Anaby D, Hand C, Bradley L et al. (2013) The effect of the environment on participation of children and youth with disabilities: a scoping review. *Disability & Rehabilitation* **35**: 1589–1598. 10.3109/09638288.2012.748840.

Antonovsky A (1996) The salutogenic model as a theory to guide health promotion. *Health Promotion International* **11**: 11–18.

Bandura A (1986) *Social Foundations of Thought and Action*. Englewood Cliffs, NJ: Prentice-Hall.

Bedell G, Coster W, Law M et al. (2013) Community participation, supports, and barriers of school-age children with and without disabilities. *Archives of Physical Medicine and Rehabilitation* **94**: 15–323. 10.1016/j.apmr.2012.09.024.

Blair SN, Morris JN (2009) Healthy hearts – and the universal benefits of being physically active: physical activity and health. *Annals of Epidemiology* **19**: 253–256. 10.1016/j.annepidem.2009.01.019.

Chatterton T (2011) *An Introduction to Thinking about 'Energy Behavior': A Multi Model Approach*. London: Department of Energy and Climate Change.

Csíkszentmihályi M (1998) *Finding Flow: The Psychology of Engagement with Everyday Life*, 1st ed. New York, NY: HarperCollins Publishers.

Darrah J, Law MC, Pollock N et al. (2011) Context therapy: a new intervention approach for children with cerebral palsy. *Developmental Medicine & Child Neurology* **53**: 615–620. 10.1111/j.1469-8749.2011.03959.x.

Dolan P, Hallsworth M, Halpern D, King D, Metcalfe R, Vlaev I (2010) *MINDSPACE: Influencing Behavior Through Public Policy*. London: C.O.a.T.I.f. Government.

Engel-Yeger B, Jarus T, Anaby D, Law M (2009) Differences in patterns of participation between youths with cerebral palsy and typically developing peers. *American Journal of Occupational Therapy* **63**: 96–104. 10.5014/ajot.63.1.96.

FHI (Norwegian Institute of Public Health) (2022) *Future Directions for Nutrition and Physical Activity Policies to Prevent NCDs Across Europe*. NIPH (fhi.no).

Gjessing B, Jahnsen RB, Strand LI, Natvik E (2018) Adaptation for participation! *Disability and Rehabilitation: Assistive Technology* **13**: 803–808. 10.1080/17483107.2017.1384075.

Heah T, Case T, McGuire B, Law M (2007) Successful participation: the lived experience among children with disabilities. *Canadian Journal of Occupational Therapy* **74**: 38–47. 10.2182/cjot.06.10.

Imms C, Granlund M, Wilson PH, Steenbergen B, Rosenbaum PL, Gordon AM (2017) Participation, both a means and an end: a conceptual analysis of processes and outcomes in childhood disability. *Developmental Medicine and Child Neurology* **59**: 16–25. 10.1111/dmcn.13237.

IvyPanda (2021) *Plato's Meno: Philosophical Dialogue* [online]. Available at: https://ivypanda.com/essays/platos-meno-philosophical-dialogue/ [Accessed 18 November 2022].

Jackson T (2005) *Motivating Sustainable Consumption: A Review of Evidence on Consumer Behavior and Behavioral Change*. London: Sustainable Development Research Network.

Kahneman D (2011) *Thinking, Fast and Slow*. London: Penguin Books Ltd.

Munro S, Lewin S, Swart T, Volmink J (2007) A review of health behavior theories: how useful are these for developing interventions to promote long-term medication adherence for TB and HIV/AIDS? *BMC Public Health* **7**: 104. 10.1186/1471-2458-7-104.

Nyquist A, Mose T, Jahnsen R (2016) Fitness, fun and friends through participation in preferred physical activities: achievable for children with disabilities? *International Journal of Disability, Development and Education* **63**: 334–356. 10.1080/1034912X.2015.1122176.

Palisano RJ, Chiarello LA, King GA, Novak I, Stoner T, Fiss A (2012) Participation-based therapy for children with physical disabilities. *Disability and Rehabilitation* **34**: 1041–1052. 10.3109/09638288.2011.628740.

Prochaska JO (1979) *Systems of Psychotherapy: A Transtheoretical Analysis*. Homewood, IL: Dorsey Press.

Rosenbaum P, Gorter JW (2012) The 'F-words' in childhood disability: I swear this is how we should think! *Child Care Health Dev* **38**: 457–463. 10.1111/j.1365-2214.2011.01338.x.

Ryan RM, Deci EL (2000) Self-determination theory and the facilitation of intrinsic motivation, social development, and well-being. *Am Psychol* **55**: 68–78. 10.1037//0003-066x.55.1.68.

Saebu M. (2011) *Physical Activity and Motivation in Young Adults With a Physical Disability: A Multidimensional Study Based on a Cross-sectional Survey and an Intervention-study*. PhD thesis, Norwegian College of Sports: Oslo.

Saebu M, Sorensen M (2011) Factors associated with physical activity among young adults with a disability. *Scand J Med Sci Sports* **21**: 730–738. 10.1111/j.1600-0838.2010.01097.x.

Saebu MS, Sorensen M, Halvari H (2013) Motivation for physical activity in young adults with physical disabilities during a rehabilitation stay: a longitudinal test of self-determination theory. *Journal of Applied Social Psychology* **43**: 612–625.

Sebire SJ, Jago R, Fox KR, Edwards MJ, Thompson JL (2013) Testing a self-determination theory model of children's physical activity motivation: a cross-sectional study. *International Journal of Behavioral Nutrition and Physical Activity* **10**: 111. 10.1186/1479-5868-10-111.

Sherrill C (2004) *Adapted Physical Activity, Recreation and Sport*, 6th ed. New York: McGraw-Hill New York.

Willis CE, Reid S, Elliott C et al. (2018) A realist evaluation of a physical activity participation intervention for children and youth with disabilities: what works, for whom, in what circumstances, and how? *BMC Pediatrics* **18**: 113. 10.1186/s12887-018-1089-8.

World Health Organization (1999) *Health Impact Assessment. Main Concepts and Suggested Approach. Gothenburg Consensus Paper*. Brussels: European Centre for Health Policy. Health Indicator Assessment. Available at: http://www.healthedpartners.org/ceu/hia/hia01/01_02_gothenburg_paper_on_hia_1999.pdf [Accessed 18 November 2022].

World Health Organization (2020) WHO Guidelines on Physical Activity and Sedentary Behaviour [online]. Available at: www.who.int/publications/i/item/9789240015128 [Accessed 18 November 2022].

CHAPTER 6

Cerebral Palsy

Désirée B Maltais, Reidun B Jahnsen,
and Maria Terese Engdahl-Høgåsen

This chapter begins with an overview of cerebral palsy (CP), including common impairments, comorbidities, and medications. Then, the different components of health-related fitness that are covered in this chapter (cardiorespiratory fitness and submaximal exercise capacity, muscular fitness, body composition, flexibility) are discussed. Definitions of these terms can be found in Chapter 2. For each component, the reasons why one might want to evaluate it are noted, followed by information on how to evaluate it and finally by either CP-specific training principles (cardiorespiratory fitness and submaximal exercise capacity, muscular fitness) or how physical activity affects the component (body composition, flexibility). The chapter concludes with suggestions for promoting a physically active lifestyle for people with CP and the voices of lived experience, an account of a person with CP becoming more fit and active.

The reader will note that the tests used to evaluate each health-related fitness component are classed as laboratory or field tests. Laboratory tests are typically used in research or specialized clinical settings, whereas field tests can be used in research, clinical, and community settings.

Throughout the chapter, when the reader is referred to resources by the statement 'see Author et al. (year)' or when article URLs are mentioned in the table legends, that means the article or document cited is freely available on the internet and the URL or other information needed to locate the article or document is found following the corresponding reference in the reference list.

WHAT IS CP?

CP is one of the most common motor disorders in children with a prevalence of between 2 and 3 per 1000 livebirths (SCPE 2000; Hollung et al. 2016). The term CP describes a group of permanent disorders of the development of movement and posture, causing limitations in movement tasks. These disorders are attributed to permanent disturbances in the developing foetal or infant brain that do not tend to worsen over time. The motor disorder of CP is often accompanied by disturbances of sensation, cognition, communication, perception, and behaviour, by epilepsy, and by secondary musculoskeletal problems (Rosenbaum et al. 2007). CP can be divided into three subgroups according to its primary effect on muscle activation: spastic (85% of individuals with CP, where muscles are stiff and the stiffness increases with the speed of movement), dyskinetic (11% of individuals with CP, where there are involuntary movements that can be slow or fast), and ataxic CP (4% of individuals with CP, where the timing of muscle activation is disturbed) (SCPE 2000; Hollung et al. 2016). The spastic form can affect one side of the body (53%) or both sides (45%) (Hollung et al. 2016). The severity (functional impact) of CP can be classified according to its impact on various functions, such as maintaining a specific position (i.e. sitting) and moving around (i.e. walking) (Gross Motor Function Classification System, GMFCS) (Palisano et al. 2008), using the hands (Manual Ability Classification System) (Eliasson et al. 2006), and communicating (Communication Function Classification System) (Hidecker et al. 2011). All three of these classification systems use a five-level scale, where level I describes a high level of function and level V describes the lowest functional level. All three classifications have been shown to describe what they intend to describe and differences in levels have been shown to be real differences (Hollung et al. 2016). About half of individuals with CP are classed in level I according to the GMFCS (Hollung et al. 2016). The proportion of individuals with CP where there is a mild impact on function is increasing, and the proportion of those with CP where there is a significant impact on function is decreasing (Hollung et al. 2016).

COMMON IMPAIRMENTS AND COMORBIDITIES

Individuals with CP can have other issues, especially those with the more severe forms. In addition to the issues noted above, people with CP can have difficulties with feeding, swallowing, and bowel motility, poor nutrition and growth, high rates of infection, and poor hearing and vision (Shevell et al. 2009). In a Norwegian population-based study of children with CP, severely impaired vision and hearing were present in 5% and 4% of the population, respectively, while active epilepsy was present in 28%, intellectual disability in 31%, and 15% were tube fed, with 28% being severely impaired or with no speech (Andersen et al. 2008).

COMMON MEDICATIONS

Since most people with CP have a spastic subtype, and one-third have epilepsy, common medications are those used to address these conditions (anti-spastic and anti-seizure medications). Botulinum neurotoxin A injections (BoNT-A) are used focally in spastic muscles to temporarily reduce the spasticity with the goal being to prevent or limit movement and pain issues by maintaining or increasing range of motion in joints at risk of reduced movement and deformities (Boyd and Hays 2001). BoNT-A injections to muscles in the calf are nearly always combined with use of ankle–foot orthoses (a brace over the calf and foot) and a period of intensive training to learn to use the new possibilities of movement.

Baclofen is a medication that acts at the level of the spinal cord to reduce spasticity globally. It can be given by mouth or from a pump that is placed under the skin at the level of the abdomen. In this latter method, the drug is more directly delivered to the spinal cord and thus less medication is needed, and there can be fewer side effects such as sleepiness (Hasnat and Rice 2015).

Chapter 3 describes epilepsy medication and other medications that could be used to treat the medical issues that can accompany CP. If the child or adult with CP has heart or lung issues or other underlying medical conditions, it is important that they are seen by a physician before they undergo exercise testing or start to increase physical activity or start an intense exercise programme, in order to ensure that they can do this safely.

CARDIORESPIRATORY FITNESS AND SUBMAXIMAL EXERCISE CAPACITY

Why Evaluate the Cardiorespiratory Fitness and Submaximal Exercise Capacity of People With CP?

The definitions of cardiorespiratory fitness and submaximal exercise capacity, the difference between children and adults, and the importance of these components of fitness to health and functioning in general are reviewed in Chapter 2. This information also applies to people with CP. For example, typically developing children who have better cardiorespiratory fitness are also those with better heart and cardiovascular health as they age (Ruiz et al. 2009; Henriksson et al. 2020). If they improve their cardiorespiratory fitness, they also show an improvement in later heart health (Ruiz et al. 2009). Since children with CP have, as a group, lower cardiorespiratory fitness than their peers who are typically developing (Verschuren et al. 2010a; Balemans et al. 2013), they may be at greater risk for poorer heart health as they age.

An evaluation of cardiorespiratory fitness can therefore provide people with CP, their families, clinicians, or researchers, an indication of whether it is low or not and therefore whether it may be relevant to improve cardiorespiratory fitness to help reduce risks for poor heart health in the future. It might also be useful to evaluate cardiorespiratory fitness if a person with CP or a caregiver has noted that the person physically tires more easily than in the past after physical activities such as running or walking or manually propelling a wheelchair. Test results can help to determine if a reduction in cardiorespiratory fitness might explain, at least in part, the change. An evaluation of cardiorespiratory fitness can also be repeated to evaluate changes over time or following an intervention. A test of submaximal exercise capacity might be chosen if a test of cardiorespiratory fitness (which is generally a test to exhaustion) is not feasible for safety or practical reasons. For submaximal exercise capacity tests that use a functional activity such as walking or propelling a manual wheelchair, the test might also be used to evaluate the functional activity itself, meaning a better score would indicate improved capacity to perform the task. This could be useful again if one is interested in changes over time or following an intervention or if there is concern that the capacity of the person to perform the functional activity has decreased over time.

How to Evaluate the Cardiorespiratory Fitness and Submaximal Exercise Capacity of People With CP

The following section provides information about evaluating the cardiorespiratory fitness and submaximal exercise capacity of people with CP. Examples of specific tests recommended by experts in the field for children (Verschuren and Balemans 2015) and adults with CP (Lennon et al. 2015) and references to test directions can be found in Table 6.1. Table 6.1 also includes information on whether the test is a laboratory or field test and the appropriate age and physical ability level for each test. Given the very limited movement abilities of children and adults functioning in GMFCS level V, a formal evaluation of cardiorespiratory and sub-maximal capacity is not feasible for them. Instead, their general mobility and movement skills can be evaluated and tracked overtime using tests such as the Gross Motor Function Measure (Russell et al. 1989, 2000, 2021; https://canchild. ca/en/resources/44-gross-motor-function-measure-gmfm).

Laboratory Tests

The basic methods of performing laboratory tests to evaluate cardiorespiratory fitness are described in Chapter 2. Given that children and adults with CP may have difficulty moving, the laboratory tests used for these individuals usually require less absolute effort at the beginning, and the level of effort may increase more slowly as the test goes along. If the individual has a great deal of difficulty moving, or if they cannot tolerate a mask or mouth-piece, then a laboratory test to directly measure cardiorespiratory fitness may not be feasible, and a clinical test of cardiorespiratory endurance or of submaximal capacity may be a feasible option. Certain safety issues are described in Chapter 3. One additional safety issue would be to ensure that the individual is correctly and properly supported during the tests to avoid injury. For safety reasons, and to ensure the tests are properly performed, the individual being tested must be able to follow simple directions.

Table 6.1 Cardiorespiratory fitness and submaximal exercise capacity tests for people with cerebral palsy (CP)

Test	Mode	Target group	Supplementary information	References
Laboratory tests of cardiorespiratory fitness				
Progressive Maximal Cycle Ergometer Test	Cycling	Children ≥6y GMFCS levels I–III	Must be able to pedal consistently at 60–70 RPM. Starting load against which the child pedals individually determined; load increase each minute based on height, GMFCS classification.	Brehm et al. (2014)*
Graded Exercise Test	Cycling	Adults GMFCS levels I–II	Starting load is 20W; load increase is 10W, 15W, or 20W, depending upon cycling ability.	De Groot et al. (2012b)*
Graded Arm Exercise Test	Arm cranking	Children ≥7y GMFCS levels III–IV	Must be able to arm-crank consistently at 40–60 RPM; starting load is 0W (no load); load increase each minute is 8W.	Verschuren et al. (2013a)*
Field tests of cardiorespiratory fitness				
GMFCS level-specific 10m shuttle run tests:	Walking, running	SRT-I, SRT-II: 6–20y SRT-III:	Separate testing protocols for each GMFCS level (I–III).	Verschuren et al. (2006)*
SRT-I, SRT-II, SRT-III		Children ≥7y	Reference values available for SRT-I and SRT-II which allow one to compare the results of a given child, young person, or young adult with CP to the results for a group of individuals of the same sex, GMFCS level, and height.	Verschuren et al. (2010a)** Verschuren et al. (2011)*
10-m shuttle ride test	Propelling a manual wheelchair	Children ≥7y GMFCS levels III–IV	A variation of the 10-m shuttle run test for children who propel a manual wheelchair throughout at least part of their day.	Verschuren et al. (2013a)*
Test of submaximal exercise capacity				
Six-minute walk test	Walking	People ≥4y GMFCS levels I–III	The Thomson et al. (2008) protocol is especially suitable for young children with CP.	Thomson et al. (2008)*
Six-minute push test	Propelling a manual wheelchair	Children ≥4y GMFCS levels III–IV	The test can also be used with children functioning in GMFCS level II who walk without aids but who also propel a wheelchair through part of the day.	Verschuren et al. (2013a)*

Mode: type of activity performed. Gross Motor Function Classification System (GMFCS) levels I–III: people functioning in GMFCS levels I–III (walk with or without walking aids). GMFCS levels I–II: people functioning in GMFCS levels I–II (walk without walking aids). GMFCS levels III–IV: people functioning in GMFCS levels III–IV (use walking aids or a wheelchair). SRT: shuttle run test. References are for articles containing test instructions (*) or reference values for comparison purposes (**). Article URLs are found in the chapter reference list. Laboratory tests are typically used in research settings or specialized clinical settings that require a measurement with a great deal of precision, otherwise field tests can be used. These latter tests can be carried out by researchers, clinicians, and other physical activity professionals. Tests are also designed for a specific target group to ensure the person performing the test has the physical abilities to perform the test correctly.

Field Tests

The most commonly used field tests of cardiorespiratory fitness are shuttle tests, the principles of which can be found in Chapter 2. These tests can be performed running, walking, or using a wheelchair depending on the individual's abilities. A 6-minute test performed walking or using a wheelchair are the most commonly used submaximal tests. The principles of these tests are also described in Chapter 2. As for laboratory tests, certain safety issues are described in Chapter 3. One additional safety issue would be to ensure that the individual is not at risk of falling if a walking or running test is performed. This may mean following the individual closely. For safety reasons, and to ensure the tests are properly performed, the individual must be able to follow simple directions as is noted above for the laboratory tests.

CP-Specific Training Principles for Cardiorespiratory Fitness

Training to improve cardiorespiratory fitness can be undertaken as part of a healthy lifestyle, for specific reasons when it is found to be low such as to reduce the risk for poor cardiovascular health with age (Ruiz et al. 2009), or to improve endurance during activities such as walking, running, or propelling a manual wheelchair.

The general guidelines found in Chapter 2 for the frequency (how often), intensity (level of effort), time (how long for a given session), and type of activity are often appropriate for individuals with CP. Training programmes that follow these guidelines can result in an improvement in cardiorespiratory fitness (Verschuren et al. 2016; Ryan et al. 2017) and possibly a slight improvement in simple gross motor functions (i.e. standing, walking, running) (Ryan et al. 2017). Longer training programmes (up to 9 months) may be more beneficial than shorter programmes (Maltais et al. 2014). What is most important for the individual with CP who wishes to engage in cardiorespiratory fitness training is that the training programme is safe and that it can be done over the long-term to avoid losing the gains as the body will adapt over time to a reduced level of physical activity if the training programme is discontinued. Thus, the training programme and its context need to be acceptable, feasible, and interesting for the individual. Clinicians and physical activity professionals with experience with physical activity and exercise for individuals with CP can help the child or adult with CP determine the right activity for them. The above-mentioned safety guidelines for evaluation of cardiorespiratory fitness also apply to training. The following are some additional training guidelines for those with CP.

Frequency

A frequency of three to five times per week is a good start. If three times a week seems too much at the beginning, the individual can start at twice a week working up to more frequent sessions.

Intensity

Also, as noted above, there are guidelines for intensity or the level of effort in Chapter 2. One can also use a more practical method of gauging the level of effort. To start, the individual can simply walk or wheel (or do whatever they have decided as their activity) at a level of effort where they can talk but not sing. The level of effort can then increase over the weeks. To gauge progressively increasing levels of effort, one can use a simple perceived level of exertion scale (https://www.physio-pedia.com/Borg_Rating_Of_Perceived_Exertion), with the first increase to 12 on the scale (felt as between 'a light and somewhat hard effort'), moving over time to a 16 on the scale (felt as between 'hard or heavy and very hard effort') (Maltais 2016). Higher levels of intensity, if desired, should be done in consultation with and under the supervision of a clinician and physical activity professional as noted above.

Time

There are no CP-specific adaptations to the duration of a given session, other than that sometimes sessions may have to start out shorter than is recommended because of the person's ability level. It is important to increase the session duration over time in a manner that is tolerable to the individual and that keeps the activity fun and interesting.

Type

The type of activity to train cardiorespiratory fitness is that which uses the large muscle groups – activities such as walking, running, wheeling, cycling, or swimming. Swimming is preferable if the individual has joint pain (Maltais 2016).

For individuals with more limited movement capacity who function in GMFCS level IV, the time and frequency of the above training guidelines may remain appropriate, but the intensity and the type of activity may not. For some children or adults who do not walk or walk only for very short distances with extensive support at the trunk (GMFCS level IV), light-intensity physical activity (where they can still sing as well as talk if they are verbal) may be the most feasible. The type of activity should vary and not all activity should be in their wheelchair. Activities on a mat or in a swimming pool can be considered, with the goals of having the individual use as many of their large muscle groups as possible. Activities in a swimming pool may be of interest given that people with CP can often more easily move in the water as the water supports part of their body weight (Maltais 2016).

People Functioning in GMFCS Level V

Since children and adults functioning in GMFCS level V have very limited ability to move, training to specifically target cardiorespiratory fitness is not feasible for them. However, they can still engage in general physical activity according to their abilities as part of a healthy lifestyle. Thus, one can also respect the time and frequency guidelines for the people functioning in the other GMFCS levels. Physical activities can be performed in their wheelchair and outside of their wheelchair. As much as is feasible, physical activities should be performed outside of their wheelchair, and postures other than sitting should be considered to provide opportunity for varied movements. The individual should always be comfortable and well supported. Supported side-lying or supported lying on the back with the upper back and head propped up or supported lying on the back in a heated pool can be considered (the latter with attention so as not to affect breathing). Voluntary movement of any kind that does not cause pain should be encouraged during the physical activity sessions (Maltais 2016).

MUSCULAR FITNESS (MUSCLE STRENGTH AND MUSCLE ENDURANCE)

Why Evaluate the Muscular Fitness of People With CP?

The importance of muscular fitness (muscle strength and muscle endurance) to overall health as described in Chapter 2 also applies to individuals with CP. Of note is that poorer muscular fitness in children is associated with an increased risk profile for cardiovascular diseases in the future (García-Hermoso et al. 2019). These risks may be greater for those with CP given they have lower levels of muscle strength (Wiley and Damiano 1998; Dekkers et al. 2020; Eken et al. 2020) and endurance (Parker et al. 1992; de Groot et al. 2012a) than their typically developing peers.

Thus, as with cardiorespiratory fitness, an evaluation of muscular fitness can provide people with CP, their families, clinicians, or researchers, an indication of whether or not it is low and therefore whether it may be relevant to improve muscular fitness to help reduce risks for poor cardiovascular health in the future. It might also be useful to evaluate the leg muscle strength of people with CP who are experiencing increasing difficulties with walking, to determine if muscle weakness could explain, at least in part, this change (Damiano and Abel 1998), especially for adults who are sedentary (Ando and Ueda 2000). For people with CP who are noticing increased fatigue along with difficulty walking, an evaluation of muscle endurance could be useful to help determine if low muscle endurance could be contributing to these changes (Eken et al. 2016). Should it be decided that an intervention to improve muscle strength or endurance or both is required, the tests can be performed again after the intervention to determine its effect.

In addition, muscle strength testing may be used to screen for muscle weakness in adults with CP who have symptoms of cervical spinal stenosis (narrowing of the bony passages for the spinal cord and spinal nerve roots). With this condition, people often note decreasing ability to use the arms or legs (which can be due to increasing muscle weakness and decreasing motor control) along with new neck pain and possibly new problems controlling the bowels or bladder (Hung et al. 2020). A referral to the person's physician is usually recommended in this situation (Hung et al. 2020).

How to Evaluate the Muscular Fitness (Muscle Strength and Muscle Endurance) of People With CP

The following section provides information about evaluating the muscular fitness of people with CP. Examples of specific tests along with references to test directions when available can be found in Table 6.2. The table also includes information on the appropriate age and physical ability level for each test. As with cardiorespiratory fitness, the very limited movement abilities of children and adults functioning in GMFCS level V, means a formal evaluation of muscular fitness is not feasible for them and instead their general mobility and movement skills can be evaluated using a test such as the Gross Motor Function Measure (Russell et al. 1989, 2000, 2021; https://canchild.ca/en/resources/44-gross-motor-function-measure-gmfm).

Laboratory Tests

Muscle strength can be measured with an isokinetic dynamometer (Chen et al. 2012; de Groot et al. 2012b). This is a device that allows muscle strength to be measured throughout the range of motion at a pre-set, constant speed (Baltzopoulos and Kellis 1998). The limb is supported during testing by attachments to the machine; for children a special attachment may be needed to accommodate their shorter limbs (Gaul 1995). A practice session is often recommended so the individual learns what is required of them (Baltzopoulos and Kellis 1998). Usually the test is performed two to four times for each muscle group evaluated to ensure a maximal effort without fatigue (Gaul 1995). Speeds will be lower for those with CP (e.g. 180° per second) (Patikas et al. 2006). This test requires the individual to be able to follow simple directions and not have deformities that would make positioning in the device painful or difficult. **Muscle endurance** can be measured using the Wingate Anaerobic test, as described in Chapter 2. The test requires the individual to be able to follow simple directions and not have any medical conditions that would prevent a short burst of high-intensity exercise.

Field Tests

Muscle strength, with the exception of calf muscle strength, can be measured in people with CP with sufficient control of muscle activation using a device called a hand-held dynamometer (Ferland et al. 2012). In this case, it is the maximum force produced by the muscle at a specific position that is measured (i.e. maximal isometric muscle strength). Use of the device requires special training, and one has to keep using the device to maintain skills. Thus, it is most often used by physical therapists in a clinical setting as opposed to educators or physical activity leaders in the community. Whether the test can be used with a given individual for a given muscle group sometimes requires a pre-test to determine feasibility. The test also requires the individual to be able to follow simple directions. **Calf muscle strength** can be estimated in children with CP who can follow simple directions using the Unilateral Heel Rise Test (Ferland et al. 2012) as developed by Yocum et al. (2010). Briefly, the participant stands facing a wall,

Table 6.2 Muscular fitness (muscle strength and muscle endurance) tests for people with cerebral palsy (CP)

Test	Mode	Target group	Supplementary information	References
Laboratory test of muscle strength				
Isokinetic dynamometry	Joint moves through full range of motion at a constant pre-set speed	≥5y GMFCS levels I–III	Limb supported by attachments to a special device. May not be feasible for people with limb deformities.	Chen et al. (2012); de Groot et al. (2012b)
Laboratory tests of muscle endurance				
20-sec Wingate cycle test	Cycling	Children ≥7y GMFCS levels I–III	Testing protocol individualized somewhat based on the abilities of the child.	Dallmeijer et al. (2013)*
Arm-cranking Wingate Anaerobic test	Arm cranking	Children ≥7y GMFCS levels III–IV	Testing protocol individualized somewhat based on the abilities of the child.	Verschuren et al. (2013b)*
Wingate cycling test	Cycling	Adults GMFCS levels I–II	Testing protocol individualized somewhat based on the abilities of the adult.	De Groot et al. (2012b)*
Field tests of muscle strength				
Hand-held dynamometry	Joint held in a pre-set position	People ≥4y GMFCS levels I–III	Feasibility for a given muscle may depend upon the person's movement abilities involving that muscle. Reference values may help to determine muscle weakness by comparing the child's results with the values for typically developing children of the same sex and similar age.	Hébert et al. (2015)***
Unilateral heel rise test	Standing	Children ≥6y GMFCS levels I–II	Measures calf muscle strength. Feasibility may depend upon the person's movement abilities involving the muscle.	Yocum et al. (2010)

(Continued)

Table 6.2 Continued

Test	Mode	Target group	Supplementary information	References
Field tests of muscle endurance				
Muscle Power Sprint Test (for leg muscles)	Fast walking, running	People 7–20y GMFCS levels I–II	Reference values allow one to compare the results of a given child, young person, or young adult with CP to the results for a group of individuals of the same sex and height.	Verschuren et al. (2007)* Verschuren et al. (2010b)**
Muscle Power Sprint Test (for arm muscles)	Propelling a manual wheelchair	Children ≥7y GMFCS levels III–IV	A variation of the Muscle Power Sprint Test for children who propel a manual wheelchair throughout at least part of their day.	Verschuren et al. (2013b)*

Mode: type of activity performed. Gross Motor Function Classification System (GMFCS) levels I–III: people functioning in GMFCS levels I–III (walk with or without walking aids). GMFCS levels I–II: people functioning in GMFCS levels I–II (walk without walking aids). GMFCS levels III–IV: people functioning in GMFCS levels III–IV (use walking aids or a wheelchair). References are for articles containing test instructions (*) or reference values for comparison purposes (**) or both (***). Article URLs are found in the chapter reference list. For the unilateral heal rise test, details on test instructions are contained in the text. Laboratory tests are typically used in research settings or specialized clinical settings that require a measurement with a great deal of precision, otherwise field tests can be used. These latter tests can be carried out by researchers, clinicians, and other physical activity professionals. Tests are also designed for a specific target group to ensure the person performing the test has the physical abilities to perform the test correctly, but in some cases a pre-test may need to be performed to ensure feasibility of the tests for a given individual.

supporting themselves on the wall with their fingertips. Then they bend the knee of the non-tested leg to clear the foot off the floor. A maximum heel rise (rising up on toes) with the other leg (the tested leg) is done. The evaluator then points a laser on the wall to use as a target (50% of the vertical distance of the maximum heel rise). The individual then performs as many heel rises as they can at a pace of 2 seconds per rise, making the laser on the wall disappear each time. The test ends if two heel rises in a row are not successful. This means the pace is not kept up, the height is not sufficient (laser target does not disappear), the other foot touches the floor, or the individual bends forward on the wall (supporting with more than the finger tips). The score is the number of successful heel rises. **Muscle endurance** can be evaluated with the Muscle Power Sprint Test. The test requires the individual to be able to follow simple directions and not have any medical conditions that would prevent them from performing short bursts of high intensity exercise. If the individual is at risk of falling during a walking or running test, an assistant may need to follow the individual closely.

CP-Specific Training Principles for Muscular Fitness

Training to improve muscular fitness can be undertaken as part of a healthy lifestyle or for specific reasons when it is found to be low such as to reduce the risk for poor cardiovascular health with age (García-Hermoso et al. 2019). Training specifically to address reduced leg muscle strength may also be undertaken in people with CP who walk as part of a programme to improve walking speed, walking balance, and overall mobility (Merino-Andrés et al. 2022). Training specifically to address reduced leg muscle endurance may be undertaken in people with CP who walk and who have increased physical fatigue and difficulty walking (Eken et al. 2016). Similarly, individuals with increasing difficulty and fatigue when propelling a manual wheelchair may also wish to engage in arm muscle strength and endurance training.

Note that for children and adults with CP functioning in GMFCS level V, the goal is that they engage in general physical activity according to their abilities as part of a healthy lifestyle as training for muscular fitness is not feasible. The guidelines for general physical activity for this group can be found at the end of the cardiorespiratory fitness training section.

Muscle Strength-Specific Training Principles

The muscle strength training principles for children and adults as covered in Chapter 2 also apply to many individuals with CP. People with CP who can strength train in the traditional manner can improve their strength (Verschuren et al. 2016; Ryan et al. 2017). As with cardiorespiratory fitness training, what is most important for the individual with CP who wishes to improve muscle strength is that the training programme is safe and that it can be done over the long term. Thus, the training programme and its context need to be acceptable, feasible, and interesting for the individual. Clinicians and physical activity professionals with experience with physical activity and exercise for individuals with CP can help the child or adult with CP determine if the general principles are appropriate, or if they need to be adapted. This might be more rest time, smaller starting weights and smaller increases in the weight over time, different kinds of equipment to train with, or adapted methods of training. The programme should be supervised to ensure the training is performed correctly for optimum results and to avoid injury. Adults or older adolescents with CP who have experience with strength training may wish to consult a professional and determine with them the level of supervision that is needed.

For some children or adults who walk using a walking aid (GMFCS level III) or who do not walk or only walk for very short distances with extensive support at the trunk (GMFCS level IV), standard muscle strength training may not be appropriate. Instead of using weights or weight machines, the load can be body weight. In these cases, there may need to be trial and error to determine the most appropriate activity, number of repetitions, and rest duration between sets. Supervision is likely required for safety, that is to ensure the activity can be done correctly to prevent injury. In some cases, physical assistance for each repetition may be needed. For this reason, a professional with experience in strength training for people with CP should develop the programme with the individual (and caregiver if there is one) and supervise it until they feel it can be supervised by another assistant (e.g. family member or a trained physical activity leader in the community). Here are some suggestions of activities to train *arm* muscles. It is important that the activities be performed as controlled movements that do not cause pain. If that is not the case, then the activity in question is not appropriate for the individual.

- Lie on the stomach with a pillow under the hips to protect the back. Raise up on the arms. Relax. Repeat to fatigue for a set.
- Start on elbows and knees on a mat. Straighten the arms as much as possible. Relax. Repeat to fatigue for a set.
- Pull to stand from a sitting on a bench. Sit back down. Repeat to fatigue for a set.

Here are some suggestions of activities to train *leg* muscles. Again, it is important that the activities only be performed if they can be done as controlled movements that do not cause pain.

- Pull to stand from sitting on a bench, pushing extra hard with the legs and using the arms as little as possible.
- Climb stairs, pushing as much as possible with the legs, and using the arms as little as possible. Each step can be considered a repetition. If necessary to ensure the activity can be performed in a controlled manner and thus safety, an assistant can help support the individual. Should the activity be very challenging, the individual can repeatedly climb up and down one or two steps rather than a flight of stairs.

Muscle Endurance-Specific Training Principles

In general, the training principles as laid out in Chapter 2 apply to people with CP. As with strength training, adaptations may be needed for those with more limited movement capacity (thus the same types of activities as used for strength training can be used for endurance training if done very quickly). Very little is known about the effects of muscle endurance training alone in CP. However, muscle endurance along with the ability to engage in everyday physical activities (participation) does improve for people with CP who can engage in a mixed training programme that follows the training guidelines for cardiorespiratory fitness, muscle strength, and muscle endurance (Ryan et al. 2017).

BODY COMPOSITION

Why Evaluate the Body Composition of People With CP?

Chapter 2 provides a description of body composition, especially body fat (body adiposity) and its importance for health, including heart health. This importance holds true for people with CP. In addition, adults with CP have a higher prevalence of diseases associated with higher levels of body fat (Ryan et al. 2014).

Thus, an evaluation of body composition can provide people with CP, their families, clinicians, or researchers, an indication of whether the person is overweight or obese and therefore whether it may be relevant to intervene to improve body composition to reduce risks for diseases such as cardiovascular disease. Similarly for people with CP who have feeding problems, an evaluation of body composition can be recommended to determine if changes to their diet are required to meet their energy requirements. Finally, should it be decided that an intervention to improve body composition is required, the tests can be performed again after the intervention to determine its effect.

How to Evaluate the Body Composition of People With CP

The following section provides information about evaluating the body composition of people with CP. Examples of specific tests are given. Directions are also provided for a commonly used field test of body composition (a measure of waist circumference) as well as references to help in interpreting the test results. Body composition tests are passive so the person's physical capacities are less relevant than when testing for cardiorespiratory fitness, submaximal exercise capacity, or muscular endurance. Instead, it is important to ensure the person is as comfortable and physically supported as needed during the test. Some ability to follow simple directions is helpful as the person needs to remain somewhat still during these tests.

Laboratory Tests

The criterion standard, dual-energy X-ray absorptiometry is recommended for people with CP (Snik and Roos 2021). Skinfold measurement and bioelectrical impedance analysis are not recommended for measuring body composition in a given individual with CP (Snik and Roos 2021). They are, however, useful for research studies where one is looking at differences between groups (Snik and Roos 2021).

Children with CP tend to have their body fat distributed differently than typically developing children; that is, their fat appears to be found more in the abdomen and muscle tissue than under the skin (Whitney et al. 2019). This makes the waist circumference measurement the preferred field test of body composition. The individual with CP should be measured lying on their back (Benner et al. 2019). CP-specific cut points for determining overweight and obese status do not yet exist, so one can use those for the general population for an estimate. For children, one can use the following charts to determine what centile the waist circumference is closest to given the child's age and sex (waist percentiles [centiles] for boys 5–19 years old: https://cpeg-gcep.net/sites/default/files/upload/bookfiles/WC_M_Dec2015.pdf; waist percentile [centiles] for girls 5–19 years old https://cpeg-gcep.net/sites/default/files/upload/bookfiles/WC_F_Dec2015.pdf). A centile of 50 would mean 50% of children have a waist circumference below the child's value. A child could be considered obese if their waist circumference is at or above the 93rd centile for their age and sex (Sharma et al. 2015). They could be considered overweight if it is or above the 75th centile (but not at or above the 93rd) (Sharma et al. 2015).

For adults, the criterion is waist circumference itself (Ross et al. 2020). Obesity is defined as a waist circumference of 105cm or more for females and 110cm or more for males. Overweight for females is defined as 90cm or more (not at or above 105cm) and for males it is 100cm or more (not at or above 110cm).

Effects of Physical Activity on the Body Composition of People With CP

Body composition does not appear to change with an exercise programme alone for children with CP (van den Berg-Emons et al. 1998). This speaks to the complex nature of body composition and the need for a more holistic approach that considers physical activity and nutrition (McPherson et al. 2016). The individual with CP who wishes to address body composition issues may wish to consult with professionals in physical activity and nutrition with experience with individuals with CP.

FLEXIBILITY

Why Evaluate the Flexibility of People With CP?

A definition of flexibility and its relevance to function in general are described in Chapter 2. The impact of flexibility on function may be even greater in people with CP because they usually have reduced flexibility involving both the arms and legs (Christensen 2020). According to a recent review (Christensen 2020), depending on where the lack of flexibility is found, it can be associated with: (1) the ball of the hip being less well seated in its socket, (2) the development of osteoarthritis over time, and

(3) difficulties walking and overall poorer mobility. Furthermore, flexibility appears to decrease over time for people with CP (Nordmark et al. 2009; Klingels et al. 2018), meaning the negative impact of a lack of flexibility may increase with ageing. Whether or not a given muscle group is at risk for reduced flexibility depends upon the movement issues and movement patterns of the individual. In general, the muscles at most risk of losing flexibility for people with CP are: (1) the muscles of the shoulder that bring the arms in towards the chest, (2) the muscles that bend the elbow and wrist (down towards the forearm), and thumb and fingers (towards the palm), (3) the muscles of the hip that bring the legs together, (4) the muscles that bend the hips and knees, and (5) the calf muscles that point the foot downward.

Flexibility of the muscles most at risk for reduced flexibility for a given person with CP should be regularly evaluated as the individual with CP ages and especially if movement ability is decreasing over time. In this way it can be determined if an intervention is required. Should it be decided that an intervention to improve flexibility is required, the tests can be performed again after the intervention to determine its effect.

How to Evaluate the Flexibility of People With CP

The following section provides information about evaluating the flexibility of people CP. Examples of specific tests are given. General directions are also provided for commonly used field tests (goniometry and inclinometry). As with body composition tests, flexibility tests are passive, so the person's physical capacities are less relevant than when testing for cardiorespiratory fitness, submaximal exercise capacity, or muscular endurance. In general, these tests are performed by the evaluator, the person does not move themselves. Thus, the ability to follow simple directions is less relevant than the ability to collaborate with the tester and not resist the movements. To help with collaboration, it is important that the person is comfortable and physically supported as needed during the test.

LABORATORY TEST

Electrogoniometers can be used for people with CP (Graham et al. 2000; Francisco-Martínez et al. 2021).

FIELD TESTS

A goniometer or an inclinometer is often used with people with CP, typically in a clinical setting (Maltais et al. 2019; Christensen 2020). To use a goniometer, both the stationary and mobile arms and the axis of movement must be lined up with the appropriate points on the body (anatomical landmarks). The devices give an angle measurement. An inclinometer also gives an angle measure. In this case, one body segment remains stationary in a pure vertical or horizontal position (checked by the inclinometer) and the other is moved and its tilt relative to the line of gravity is measured by placing the inclinometer on the segment at a specific location. Both methods require an experienced evaluator and can be affected by the behaviour of the individual being measured or by motor control issues. The choice of the device can depend on personal experience and preference.

Effects of Physical Activity on Flexibility of People With CP

In general it is recommended flexibility exercises are performed three times weekly as part of a physically active healthy lifestyle. This would hold true for individuals with CP, but flexibility exercises per se are not recommended as a method to improve flexibility (Novak et al. 2013). The typically used interventions to improve flexibility for people with CP, when it interferes with their daily functioning, are serial casting, bracing, and various types of orthopaedic surgery (Christensen 2020). However, physical activity such as regularly walking on a treadmill may reduce the stiffness in the calf muscles and improve heel strike in both children and adults with CP who walk with and without assistive devices (GMFCS levels I–III) (Willerslev-Olsen et al. 2014; Lorentzen et al. 2017). These types of programmes could be considered complementary to more invasive methods to manage flexibility issues at the ankle and could perhaps be especially used to maintain gains from these other methods. Thus, while changes were seen to maintain gains in these treadmill programmes after 4 weeks in children and 6 weeks for adults, the programme may need to be ongoing at least a few times per week after the initial period. The programme should be supervised during the initial period by a clinician or physical activity professional with experience with treadmill training for people with CP. This individual can also assess the extent of supervision needed during the treadmill walking periods and train the person who will be doing the day-to-day supervision for an ongoing programme.

Here is a summary of a training programme (Willerslev-Olsen et al. 2014) that was associated with reduced calf muscle stiffness and better foot clearance and heel strike during walking for children with CP:

- 30 minutes per day of treadmill walking for at least 1 month using the handrails.
- The 30 minutes can be accumulated throughout the day or done at one time.
- The walking speed is what is comfortable for the child and progressively increased over the 4 weeks as tolerated.
- The treadmill is on an incline that is challenging for the child but not fatiguing (at least 5%).
- The incline increases over time to remain challenging (emphasis on increasing the incline as opposed to the speed).
- While walking on the treadmill, the child practises putting the heel down first with each step.

A training programme (Lorentzen et al. 2017) that was associated with reduced calf muscle stiffness and better foot clearance and heel strike during walking for adults with CP is similar to the above protocol but with the following exceptions:

- The 30 minutes per day is consecutive.
- 6 weeks as opposed to 4 weeks may be needed to see changes.
- The speed should be challenging and increase 0.2km per hour per week.
- The incline should start at 3% to 5% and increase 1% per week.

PROMOTING A PHYSICALLY ACTIVE LIFESTYLE FOR PEOPLE WITH CP

The benefits of a physically activity lifestyle in general have been covered in part in Chapter 2 and in the present chapter for the different elements of health-related fitness. In addition, a physically activity lifestyle for people with CP is associated with improvements in spasticity (muscle stiffness), quality of life, and participation in daily life (Lai et al. 2021).

The general approach to a physically active lifestyle as discussed in Chapter 5 applies to people with CP. Methods to address specific challenges for people with CP have been covered above under the CP-specific training principles for the different elements of health-related fitness. To demonstrate the points discussed in this chapter in a real-world context, here is the story of a young dancer with CP called Sarah, who is 25 years old and in GMFCS level I.

VOICES WITH LIVED EXPERIENCE

This girl, Sarah, is quiet and careful. She is scared. Scared of falling, scared of failing. Scared because she is different. She tells herself she can't do what everyone else can, that she can't do the things she wants to. Better yet, she decides she doesn't actually want to. She decides she doesn't like sports, that she doesn't like being as active as the other kids.

Sarah was born with CP, to a degree so mild that it was barely evident. Actually, you probably wouldn't see it at all. So according to the doctors it wouldn't affect her much. Sarah would walk as well as the other kids, she would run as fast, climb as high, and smile as wide. None of the doctors ever mentioned struggling with keeping up with the others, and no one suggested regular physical therapy or any activities in particular.

Let's pause for a minute: Sarah gets a diagnosis. But what good (or perhaps harm) does that do? CP becomes a useless label. She is supposed to be 'normal', but yet she is not. Imagine how it would feel if someone took away your left arm and told you that 'You don't need it anyway. You'll be just fine'.

OK. Back to the story:

As time and childhood pass, Sarah turns out pretty much like any other kid, I guess. But she doesn't run much. She sits for hours playing quiet games. She loves her stroller, and her parents let her sit in it till she is way too old. Sarah tells herself the same lie as the doctors: 'I am just the same, I am just like them.' She tries so hard to believe it. She works so hard to prove it. Still she experiences all the differences, the struggle, and the frustration.

While the other kids don't mind walking to the local pool for their swimming lesson, she is in pain. When all the other kids learn how to swim she is still wearing arm floats. Sarah is told to do all the same things, she tries, but she feels like she's failing. Sarah, her parents, and even some of the teachers know that she has a disability, but they don't know what it means. So Sarah tells her parents she doesn't like football, that gymnastics isn't for her, that she'd rather stay at home than go hiking. She becomes Sarah, the girl that I used to know.

OK let's stop again for a minute. Sarah is being treated as if she is just like everyone else, and I guess to some extent that is ideal. She is never told she can't do what she wants, that she can't reach her highest goal. She is never looked at differently. But what about the day she realizes she actually is different? What about the day she realizes that she actually wants to do all the things she pretended she did not want to do? What about the effort she puts into being 'normal' that no one recognized?

Remember how I asked you to imagine your arm being cut off. Now, imagine it's not cut off. It is still there, just not working. To anyone else you look perfectly fine, yet I imagine you would feel pretty helpless.

We're back to the story again. Sarah is 16. Believe it or not, she has decided she wants to be a dancer. By some lucky chance she falls in love with music, with movement. For some incredible reason, and thanks to some pretty special teachers, she decides to push through the pain, through the struggle. She decides she can work hard and become good at dancing. And so she does. She becomes not only a good dancer, she becomes a great one. Except great comes in different forms, different understandings. Sarah works harder than most others. Still her greatness won't fit the 'normal' scale. So she works even harder. To the point of breakdown.

By this time, Sarah is way past knowing she is different. She has felt it every day for years. She has felt like lifting 100kg every time she balances on one leg, like she has run a marathon after every demanding routine. She knows too well that she has a disability. But there is a difference between knowing and accepting, and there is a difference between accepting and stopping trying to be normal.

At 16, Sarah spends her nights crying. Her tears come from a combination of the physical pain and exhaustion, and a deep sorrow – a sorrow that is unexplainable, incomprehensible. She wishes her left leg gone, she wishes her disability visible, she wishes everyone would see how hard she is trying. She cries and she quits. She quits her dream.

I started off telling you Sarah was a girl that I once knew. One I don't know anymore. That's because Sarah doesn't exist anymore. Because I used to be her. But I am not anymore. She was with me for many years, but now she is finally gone.

Today I dare to call myself a dancer. Today I know I would be so much more 'disabled' without the hours of training and the hard work I put into trying to become a perfect dancer. And the greatest part: today I know what a huge job I did. I know that some days I put in the same effort as an athlete just to get through a normal day.

Sarah was a scared girl. A careful girl that told herself she couldn't do things. She decided not to try at all. She would dance, but she preferred to stay in her comfort zone. Now that she is gone I can try new things. All the time. And I can be immensely proud when I ski down a hill, stand up on a surf board, or balance across a slackline. I can laugh when I fall, but I can cry when I see a 'perfect' dancer. I can try just about anything, but I can quit when I want to. I can be me. I can be Maria. Sarah is gone. And to that I owe the inspiring dancing teacher that saw my struggle, The Norwegian School of Sport Science and all the teachers that let me crawl but pushed me to run, the swimming instructor that saw me sink but dared me to swim and refused to let me quit. I owe it to my parents, who never pushed me too hard but always supported me, and to the amazing artists that showed me what dance and movement could be about. I am forever grateful for all the people that encouraged me, for who I was. Who saw my limitations, but still believed in me. The people who acknowledged my struggle.

I know now that I am disabled but mostly abled. I know I can do most things but not everything. If I could go back I would tell her that. I would tell Sarah that it is always better to try, but it is OK to fail.

Sarah is gone now. But I will never forget her.

REFERENCES

Andersen GL, Irgens LM, Haagaas I, Skranes JS, Meberg AE, Vik T (2008) Cerebral palsy in Norway: prevalence, subtypes and severity. *Eur J Paediatr Neurol* **12**: 4–13. 10.1016/j.ejpn.2007.05.001.

Ando N, Ueda S (2000) Functional deterioration in adults with cerebral palsy. *Clin Rehabil* **14**: 300–306.

Balemans AC, Van Wely L, De Heer SJ et al. (2013) Maximal aerobic and anaerobic exercise responses in children with cerebral palsy. *Med Sci Sports Exerc* **45**: 561–568. 10.1249/MSS.0b013e3182732b2f. PMID: 23034639.

Baltzopoulos V, Kellis E (1998) Isokinetic strength during childhood and adolescence. In: Van Praagh E, editor, *Pediatric Anaerobic Performance*. Champaign: Human Kinetics, pp 225–240.

Boyd RN, Hays RM (2001) Current evidence for the use of botulinum toxin type A in the management of children with cerebral palsy: a systematic review. *Eur J Neurol* **8**: pp 1–20.

Benner JL, McPhee PG, Gorter JW et al. (2019) Focus on risk factors for cardiometabolic disease in cerebral palsy: toward a core set of outcome measurement instruments. *Arch Phys Med Rehabil* **100**: 2389–2398.

Brehm MA, Balemans AC, Becher JG, Dallmeijer AJ (2014) Reliability of a progressive maximal cycle ergometer test to assess peak oxygen uptake in children with mild to moderate cerebral palsy. *Phys Ther* **94**: 121–128. **https://academic.oup.com/ptj/article/94/1/121/2735460**.

Chen CL, Lin KC, Wu CY, Ke JY, Wang CJ, Chen CY (2012) Relationships of muscle strength and bone mineral density in ambulatory children with cerebral palsy. *Osteoporos Int* **23**: 715–721.

Christensen C (2020) Flexibility in children and youth with cerebral palsy. In: Miller F, Bachrach S, Lennon N, O'Neil ME, editors, *Cerebral Palsy*. Champaign: Springer, pp 2709–2732.

Dallmeijer AJ, Scholtes VA, Brehm MA, Becher JG (2013) Test-retest reliability of the 20-sec Wingate test to assess anaerobic power in children with cerebral palsy. *Am J Phys Med Rehabil* **92**: 762–767. **https://journals.lww.com/ajpmr/Abstract/2013/09000/Test_Retest_Reliability_of_the_20_sec_Wingate_Test.4.aspx (the article is freely available on the Internet and can be located using a search engine)**.

Damiano DL, Abel MF (1998) Functional outcomes of strength training in spastic cerebral palsy. *Arch Phys Med Rehabil* **79**: 119–125.

de Groot S, Dallmeijer AJ, Bessems PJ, Lamberts ML, van der Woude LH, Janssen TW (2012a) Comparison of muscle strength, sprint power and aerobic capacity in adults with and without cerebral palsy. *J Rehabil Med* **44**: 932–938.

De Groot S, Janssen TW, Evers M, Van der Luijt P, Nienhuys KN, Dallmeijer AJ (2012b) Feasibility and reliability of measuring strength, sprint power, and aerobic capacity in athletes and non-athletes with cerebral palsy. *Dev Med Child Neurol* **54**: 647–653. **https://onlinelibrary.wiley.com/doi/epdf/10.1111/j.1469-8749.2012.04261.x**.

Dekkers KJFM, Rameckers EAA, Smeets RJEM et al. (2020) Upper extremity muscle strength in children with unilateral spastic cerebral palsy: a bilateral problem? *Phys Ther* **100**: 2205–2216.

Eken MM, Lamberts RP, Koschnick S, Du Toit J, Veerbeek BE, Langerak NG (2020) Lower extremity strength profile in ambulatory adults with cerebral palsy and spastic diplegia: norm values and reliability for hand-held dynamometry. *PM R* **12**: 573–580.

Eken MM, Houdijk H, Doorenbosch CA et al. (2016) Relations between muscle endurance and subjectively reported fatigue, walking capacity, and participation in mildly affected adolescents with cerebral palsy. *Dev Med Child Neurol* **58**: 814–821.

Eliasson AC, Krumlinde-Sundholm L, Rosblad B et al. (2006) The Manual Ability Classification System (MACS) for children with cerebral palsy: scale development and evidence of validity and reliability. *Dev Med Child Neurol* **48**: 549–554.

Ferland C, Lepage C, Moffet H, Maltais DB (2012) Relationships between lower limb muscle strength and locomotor capacity in children and adolescents with cerebral palsy who walk independently. *Phys Occup Ther Pediatr* **32**: 320–332. 10.3109/01942638.2011.631102.

Francisco-Martínez C, Prado-Olivarez J, Padilla-Medina JA et al. (2021) Upper limb movement measurement systems for cerebral palsy: a systematic literature review. *Sensors (Basel)* **26**: 7884.

García-Hermoso A, Ramírez-Campillo R, Izquierdo M (2019) Is muscular fitness associated with future health benefits in children and adolescents? A systematic review and meta-analysis of longitudinal studies. *Sports Med* **49**: 1079–1094.

Gaul CA (1995) Muscular strength and endurance. In: Docherty D, editor, *Measurement in Pediatric Exercise Science*. Champaign: Human Kinetics, pp 225–258.

Graham HK, Aoki KR, Autti-Rämö I et al. (2000) Recommendations for the use of botulinum toxin type A in the management of cerebral palsy. *Gait Posture* **11**: 67–79.

Hasnat MJ, Rice JE (2015) Intrathecal baclofen for treating spasticity in children with cerebral palsy. *The Cochrane Database of Systematic Reviews* **11**: Cd004552.

Hébert LJ, Maltais DB, Lepage C, Saulnier J, Crête M (2015) Hand-held dynamometry isometric torque reference values for children and adolescents. *Pediatr Phys Ther* **27**: 414–423. **https://www.ncbi.nlm.nih.gov/pmc/articles/PMC4581449/pdf/ppyty-27-414.pdf**.

Henriksson H, Henriksson P, Tynelius P et al. (2020) Cardiorespiratory fitness, muscular strength, and obesity in adolescence and later chronic disability due to cardiovascular disease: a cohort study of 1 million men. *Eur Heart J* **14**: 1503–1510.

Hidecker MJ, Paneth N, Rosenbaum PL et al. (2011) Developing and validating the Communication Function Classification System for individuals with cerebral palsy. *Dev Med Child Neurol* **53**: 704–710.

Hollung SJ, Vik T, Wiik R, Bakken IJ, Andersen GL (2016) Completeness and correctness of cerebral palsy diagnoses in two health registers: implications for estimating prevalence. *Dev Med Child Neuro* **59**: 402–406. 10.1111/dmcn.13341.

Hung CW, Matsumoto H, Ball JR et al. (2020) Symptomatic cervical spinal stenosis in spastic cerebral palsy. *Dev Med Child Neurol* **62**: 1147–1153.

Klingels K, Meyer S, Mailleux L et al. (2018) Time course of upper limb function in children with unilateral cerebral palsy: a five-year follow-up study. *Neural Plast* **14**: 2831342.

Lai B, Lee E, Kim Y et al. (2021) Leisure-time physical activity interventions for children and adults with cerebral palsy: a scoping review. *Dev Med Child Neurol* **63**: 162–171.

Lennon N, Thorpe D, Balemans AC et al. (2015) The clinimetric properties of aerobic and anaerobic fitness measures in adults with cerebral palsy: a systematic review of the literature. *Res Dev Disabil* **45–46**: 316–328.

Lorentzen J, Kirk H, Fernandez-Lago H et al. (2017) Treadmill training with an incline reduces ankle joint stiffness and improves active range of movement during gait in adults with cerebral palsy. *Disabil Rehabil* **39**: 987–993.

Maltais, DB (2016) Cerebral palsy. In: Moore GE, Moore GE, Durstine JL, editors, *ACSM's Exercise Management for Persons with Chronic Diseases and Disabilities*, 4th ed. Champaign, IL: Human Kinetics, pp 259–266.

Maltais DB, Ferland C, Perron M, Roy JS (2019) Reliability of inclinometer-derived passive range of motion measures in youth with cerebral palsy. *Phys Occup Ther Pediatr* **39**: 655–668.

Maltais DB, Wiart L, Fowler E, Verschuren O, Damiano DL (2014) Health-related physical fitness for children with cerebral palsy. *J Child Neurol* **29**: 1091–100.

McPherson AC, Ball GD, Maltais DB et al. (2016) A call to action: setting the research agenda for addressing obesity and weight-related topics in children with physical disabilities. *Child Obes* **12**: 59–69.

Merino-Andrés J, García de Mateos-López A, Damiano DL, Sánchez-Sierra A (2022) Effect of muscle strength training in children and adolescents with spastic cerebral palsy: a systematic review and meta-analysis. *Clin Rehabil* **36**: 4–14.

Nordmark E, Hägglund G, Lauge-Pedersen H, Wagner P, Westbom L (2009) Development of lower limb range of motion from early childhood to adolescence in cerebral palsy: a population-based study. *BMC Med* **28**: 65.

Novak I, McIntyre S, Morgan C et al. (2013) A systematic review of interventions for children with cerebral palsy: state of the evidence. *Dev Med Child Neurol* **55**: 885–910.

Palisano RJ, Rosenbaum P, Bartlett D, Livingston MH (2008) Content validity of the expanded and revised gross motor function classification system. *Developmental Medicine and Child Neurology* **50**: 744–750.

Parker DF, Carriere L, Hebestreit H, Bar-Or O (1992) Anaerobic endurance and peak muscle power in children with spastic cerebral palsy. *Am J Dis Child* **146**: 1069–1073.

Patikas D, Wolf SI, Armbrust P et al. Effects of a postoperative resistive exercise program on the knee extension and flexion torque in children with cerebral palsy: a randomized clinical trial. *Arch Phys Med Rehabil* **87**: 1161–1169.

Rosenbaum P, Paneth N, Leviton A et al. (2007) A report: the definition and classification of cerebral palsy April 2006. *Dev Med Child Neurol Suppl* **109**: 8–14.

Ross R, Neeland IJ, Yamashita S et al. (2020) Waist circumference as a vital sign in clinical practice: a consensus statement from the IAS and ICCR Working Group on Visceral Obesity. *Nat Rev Endocrinol* **16**: 177–189.

Ruiz JR, Castro-Piñero J, Artero EG et al. Predictive validity of health-related fitness in youth: a systematic review. *Br J Sports Med* **43**: 909–923.

Russell DJ, Avery LM, Rosenbaum PL et al. (2000) Improved scaling of the Gross Motor Function Measure for children with cerebral palsy. *Phys Ther* **80**: 873–885.

Russell DJ, Palisano RJ, Walter S et al. (1989) The Gross Motor Function Measure. *Dev Med Child Neurol* **31**: 341–352.

Russell DJ, Wright M, Rosenbaum PL, Avery LM, editors (2021) *Gross Motor Function Measure (GMFM-66 & GMFM-88) User's Manual 3rd Edition*. London: Mac Keith Press.

Ryan JM, Cassidy EE, Noorduyn SG, O'Connell NE (2017) Exercise interventions for cerebral palsy. *Cochrane Database Syst Rev* **6**: CD011660.

Ryan JM, Crowley VE, Hensey O, McGahey A, Gormley J (2014) Waist circumference provides an indication of numerous cardiometabolic risk factors in adults with cerebral palsy. *Arch Phys Med Rehabil* **95**: 1540–1546.

Shevell MI, Dagenais L, Hall N (2009) Comorbidities in cerebral palsy and their relationship to neurologic subtype and GMFCS level. *Neurology* **16**: 2090–2096.

Snik DAC, de Roos NM (2021) Criterion validity of assessment methods to estimate body composition in children with cerebral palsy: a systematic review. *Ann Phys Rehabil Med* **64**: 101271.

Sharma AK, Metzger DL, Daymont C, Hadjiyannakis S, Rodd CJ (2015) LMS tables for waist-circumference and waist-height ratio Z-scores in children aged 5–19 y in NHANES III: association with cardio-metabolic risks. *Pediatr Res* **78**: 723–729.

SCPE (Surveillance of Cerebral Palsy in Europe) Collaborative Group (2000) Surveillance of cerebral palsy in Europe: a collaboration of cerebral palsy surveys and registers. *Dev Med Child Neurol* **42**: 816–824.

Thompson P, Beath T, Bell J et al. (2008) Test-retest reliability of the 10-metre fast walk test and 6-minute walk test in ambulatory school-aged children with cerebral palsy. *Dev Med Child Neurol* **50**: 370–376. **https://onlinelibrary.wiley.com/doi/epdf/10.1111/j.1469-8749.2008.02048.x**.

Van den Berg-Emons RJ, Van Baak MA, Speth L, Saris WH (1998) Physical training of school children with spastic cerebral palsy: effects on daily activity, fat mass and fitness. *International Journal of Rehabilitation Research* **21**: 179–194.

Verschuren O, Balemans AC (2015) Update of the core set of exercise tests for children and adolescents with cerebral palsy. *Pediatr Phys Ther* **27**: 187–189.

Verschuren O, Bloemen M, Kruitwagen C, Takken T (2010a) Reference values for aerobic fitness in children, adolescents, and young adults who have cerebral palsy and are ambulatory. *Phys Ther* **90**: 1148–1156. **https://academic.oup.com/ptj/article/90/8/1148/2737992**.

Verschuren O, Bloemen M, Kruitwagen C, Takken T (2010b) Reference values for anaerobic performance and agility in ambulatory children and adolescents with cerebral palsy. *Dev Med Child Neurol* **52**: e222–e228. **https://onlinelibrary.wiley.com/doi/epdf/10.1111/j.1469-8749.2010.03747.x**.

Verschuren O, Bosma L, Takken T (2011) Reliability of a shuttle run test for children with cerebral palsy who are classified at Gross Motor Function Classification System level III. *Dev Med Child Neurol* **53**: 470–472. **https://onlinelibrary.wiley.com/doi/epdf/10.1111/j.1469-8749.2010.03893.x**.

Verschuren O, Ketelaar M, De Groot J, Vila Nova F, Takken T (2012) Reproducibility of two functional field exercise tests for children with cerebral palsy who self-propel a manual wheelchair. *Dev Med Child Neurol* **55**: 185–190. **https://onlinelibrary.wiley.com/doi/epdf/10.1111/dmcn.12052**.

Verschuren O, Peterson MD, Balemans AC, Hurvitz EA (2016) Exercise and physical activity recommendations for people with cerebral palsy. *Dev Med Child Neurol* **58**: 798–808.

Verschuren O, Takken T, Ketelaar M, Gorter JW, Helders PJ (2006) Reliability and validity of data for 2 newly developed shuttle run tests in children with cerebral palsy. *Phys Ther* **86**: 1107–1117. **https://academic.oup.com/ptj/article/86/8/1107/2857457**.

Verschuren O, Takken T, Ketelaar M, Gorter JW, Helders PJ (2007) Reliability for running tests for measuring agility and anaerobic muscle power in children and adolescents with cerebral palsy. *Pediatr Phys Ther* **19**: 108–115.

Verschuren O, Zwinkels M, Ketelaar M, Reijnders-van Son F, Takken T (2013a) Reproducibility and validity of the 10-meter shuttle ride test in wheelchair-using children and adolescents with cerebral palsy. *Phys Ther* **93**: 967–974. **https://academic.oup.com/ptj/article/93/7/967/2735430**.

Verschuren O, Zwinkels M, Obeid J, Kerkhof N, Ketelaar M, Takken T (2013b) Reliability and validity of short-term performance tests for wheelchair-using children and adolescents with cerebral palsy. *Dev Med Child Neurol* **55**:1129–1135. **https://onlinelibrary.wiley.com/doi/epdf/10.1111/dmcn.12214**.

Whitney DG, Gross-Richmond P, Hurvitz EA, Peterson MD (2019) Total and regional body fat status among children and young people with cerebral palsy: a scoping review. *Clin Obes* **9**: e12327.

Wiley ME, Damiano DL (1998) Lower-extremity strength profiles in spastic cerebral palsy. *Dev Med Child Neurol* **40**: 100–107.

Willerslev-Olsen M, Lorentzen J, Nielsen JB (2014) Gait training reduces ankle joint stiffness and facilitates heel strike in children with cerebral palsy. *NeuroRehabilitation* **35**: 643–655.

Yocum A, McCoy SW, Bjornson KF, Mullens P, Burton GN (2010) Reliability and validity of the standing heel-rise test. *Phys Occup Ther Pediatr* **30**:190–120.

CHAPTER 7

Developmental Coordination Disorder

Sara King-Dowling, Jeffrey D Graham, and John Cairney

This chapter begins with a description of developmental coordination disorder (DCD) that includes the diagnostic criteria. This is followed by a discussion of common impairments, comorbidities, and medications. Next, the health-related fitness components of cardiorespiratory fitness and submaximal exercise capacity, muscular fitness, body composition, and flexibility are reviewed (see Chapter 2 for definitions of these terms). For each component, the reader is provided with information on why one might wish to evaluate it, how to evaluate it, and either DCD-specific training principles (cardiorespiratory fitness and submaximal exercise capacity, muscular fitness) or a discussion about how physical activity affects the component (body composition, flexibility). The chapter ends with an overview of guidelines to promote a physically active lifestyle for people with DCD.

The reader will also note that the health-related fitness tests are classed as laboratory or field tests. Laboratory tests are often employed in research or specialized clinical contexts. Field tests are typically used in research, clinical, and community contexts. Chapter 2 provides a more detailed description of laboratory and field tests.

Throughout the chapter, when the reader is referred to resources by the statement 'see Author et al. (year)' or when article URLs are mentioned in the table legends, that means the article or document cited is freely available on the internet and the URL or other information needed to locate the article or document is found following the corresponding reference in the reference list.

WHAT IS DCD?

At its core, DCD is a neurodevelopmental disorder that affects movement, where the individual presents with motor coordination functioning well below that of their typically developing peers (American Psychiatric Association 2013). It is seen in 2% to 5% of children (Gibbs et al. 2007). It can also persist into adulthood. While currently the preferred term is DCD, over the years the condition has been referred to by other names such as 'clumsy child syndrome', 'developmental dyspraxia, or motor learning disorder, (Sugden et al. 2006).

An official diagnosis of DCD is made by a physician who must rule out other conditions that might result in similar movement difficulties. For children, these could be conditions such as cerebral palsy or muscular dystrophy. Examples of other medical conditions that must be ruled out at any age before the diagnosis is made are a brain tumour or recent head trauma. Difficulties with movement are typically defined as results on a test of motor coordination in the bottom 15th percentile (>5 years old) or the bottom 5th percentile (3–5 years old) compared to the results of typically developing peers (Blank et al. 2019). For children, an example of such a test is the Movement Assessment Battery for Children, Second Edition (MABC-2) (Henderson and Sugden 2007). To be diagnosed with DCD, the individual must also show problems in movement-based activities related to scholastics and/or problems with activities of everyday living such as tying shoelaces or other aspects of self-care, or reduced participation in sport and play (American Psychiatric Association 2013). There must also be evidence that the movement coordination problems were present in the early development period, given DCD is considered to be a 'developmental' (i.e. child-onset) condition (Henderson and Henderson 2003).

COMMON IMPAIRMENTS AND COMORBIDITIES

How the condition is manifested in an individual with DCD varies. Some individuals show difficulties in one area, such as large gross motor movements (e.g. performing a jumping jack), fine movements (e.g. writing), or balance; others show difficulties in all three areas (Wright and Sugden 1996). These difficulties are believed to be due in part to problems with planning movements and processing visuospatial information (Wilson and McKenzie 1998; Geuze 2005). For example, Wilson and colleagues (2001, 2002) have shown that children with DCD are not only slower at executing motor tasks, requiring more conscious or effortful attention to sustain movement patterns, but are also slower at imagining the execution of these tasks. Individuals with DCD also experience deficits in cognitive control (Wilson et al. 2017). This means they can have difficulty with the thinking processes that guide behaviour, including attention, self-regulation, and self-control (Miyake et al. 2000; Hofmann et al. 2012). Problems with paying attention can be a challenge when the individual with DCD is learning the rules of an activity or how to perform a new task. In children, problems with self-regulation that lead to behavioural outbursts may also affect learning. Cognitive control processes are important for overall physical and mental health throughout the lifespan (Mischel et al. 2011), including participation in physical activity (Buckley et al. 2014). Thus, these issues need to be taken into consideration by the person with DCD and those supporting their engagement in physical activities.

Overall, the difficulties experienced by people with DCD suggest that certain parts of the brain may be affected, such as the cerebellum (a structure in the back of the brain that supports coordination of movement) and parietal lobe (a lobe in the upper back part of the brain that processes information regarding temperature, taste, touch, and movement) (Zwicker et al. 2009). Although the cause or origins of the condition are still unclear and likely multi-factorial, the onset of the disorder is believed to occur in early life, before birth or possibly shortly after birth, as the brain is developing (Gubbay et al. 1975; Holsti et al. 2002).

People with DCD often have other neurodevelopmental disorders in addition to DCD, such as attention-deficit/hyperactivity disorder (ADHD), learning difficulties, or language difficulties (Zwicker et al. 2012). Some individuals may also have DCD and autism spectrum disorder (American Psychiatric Association 2013; Cairney and King-Dowling, 2015).

COMMON MEDICATIONS

Chapter 3 reviews safety considerations in general for physical activity. While there are no medications used to treat DCD per se, for individuals with DCD and ADHD, stimulant medications may be used to manage ADHD. If stimulants are used, the individual performing intense physical activity on a regular basis could be at increased risk for heart issues or heat injury (if the activity is performed in hot conditions) (Pujalte et al. 2019). Therefore, if an individual with DCD is taking stimulant medications their physician should be aware of their activities and be consulted as necessary.

CARDIORESPIRATORY FITNESS AND SUBMAXIMAL EXERCISE CAPACITY

Why Evaluate the Cardiorespiratory Fitness and Submaximal Exercise Capacity of People With DCD?

Chapter 2 presents definitions of cardiorespiratory fitness and submaximal exercise capacity, including differences in general between children and adults, and the relevance of cardiorespiratory fitness and submaximal exercise capacity to overall health and functioning. For example, typically developing children with higher levels of cardiorespiratory fitness also show a higher level of heart and cardiovascular health as they age (Ruiz et al. 2009; Henriksson et al. 2020). Furthermore, an improvement in cardiorespiratory fitness is associated with an improvement in heart health as they grow older (Ruiz et al. 2009). This information would also apply to people with DCD.

In addition, children with DCD have lower cardiorespiratory fitness than their typically developing peers (Cairney et al. 2010a; King-Dowling et al. 2018), and they show an increased risk for chronic diseases related to poor heart heath (Joshi et al. 2015). Thus, an evaluation of cardiorespiratory fitness might provide valuable information to individuals with DCD, their families, clinicians, physical activity professionals, or researchers regarding whether or not it is low and consequently whether or not it might be beneficial to improve cardiorespiratory fitness to help reduce risks for future poor heart health. It might also be helpful to evaluate cardiorespiratory fitness if the individual with DCD or a family member, teacher, or community fitness leader noticed that the individual was having difficulty participating in physical activities that required good cardiorespiratory fitness (e.g. basketball, cross-country running, football, swimming). Test results could help to ascertain if low cardiorespiratory fitness was responsible for at least part of the difficulty, in addition to their motor coordination issues. A test of submaximal exercise capacity might be chosen if a test of cardiorespiratory fitness (which is generally a test to exhaustion) is not feasible for safety or practical reasons. Repeating either type of test can be used to determine changes over time or after an intervention.

How to Evaluate the Cardiorespiratory Fitness and Submaximal Exercise Capacity of People With DCD

The following section provides information about evaluating the cardiorespiratory fitness and submaximal exercise capacity of people with DCD.

Laboratory Tests

The same laboratory tests used with typically developing children and adults as described in Chapter 2 tend to also be appropriate for those with DCD. The exact test used may depend upon the question. For example, if the question is a research or medical question that involves taking blood from the arm during or after the test, it may be more feasible to use a cycling test as the arms are relatively still during this type of test. If the question relates to cardiorespiratory fitness for running activities, it may be more appropriate to use a treadmill test where the person runs on the treadmill. If using a cycling test, it may be prudent, first, to determine if the individual can maintain cycling at the required cadence (speed) as younger children with DCD, and people with DCD with more severe motor challenges may find this difficult. If this is the case, a treadmill test may be the more feasible option overall, if a laboratory test is required, as the speed is dictated by movement of the treadmill belt. If an individual has substantial balance difficulties, holding on to the handrails may be necessary during the treadmill test.

Field Tests

The most feasible field test to estimate cardiorespiratory fitness in people with DCD may be the 20m shuttle run test as described in Chapter 2. When carrying out this test with people with DCD, especially children under 8 years old, someone may have to run with them to help them maintain an appropriate pace. See De Miguel-Etayo et al. (2014) for reference values in percentiles for typically developing males and females aged 6 to 9 years old. See Ortega et al. (2011) for similar reference values but for young people aged 13 to 17 years old. These values can be used to determine if the child or young person has low cardiorespiratory fitness. A percentile of 50 for a given child would mean 50% of children or young people of the same age and sex have a cardiorespiratory fitness value below the child or young person's value. Submaximal exercise capacity can be evaluated with the 6-minute walk test, also described in Chapter 2. See Li et al. (2007) for reference values in percentiles for males and females aged 7 to 16 years old for the 6-minute walk test. In this case, the values should be used as an estimate given there may be relevant differences not accounted for in the reference values, such as the country of origin (Cacau et al. 2016).

DCD-Specific Training Principles for Cardiorespiratory Fitness

Cardiorespiratory fitness training can be done as part of a healthy lifestyle. It can also be undertaken if it is found to be low to decrease the risk for poor cardiovascular health with age (Ruiz et al. 2009) or to improve endurance during activities such as playing basketball, cross-country running, football, or swimming.

The guidelines in Chapter 2 for frequency (how often), intensity (level of effort), and time (how long for a given session) are overall appropriate for people with DCD. As shown by Farhat et al. (2015), an 8-week training program of walking, running, climbing, and jumping activities was successful at improving cardiorespiratory fitness in children with DCD. The choice of the type of activity or activities for a given individual should be focused on their abilities and interests to help ensure that the regular performance of the activity can be sustained over time so gains are maintained, since the body will adapt over time to reduced levels of physical activity should regular performance of the activity cease. For children, the involvement of parents and teachers can provide additional support and help to also sustain the gains made (Sugden and Chambers 2003; Smits-Engelsman et al. 2013; Camden et al. 2015).

MUSCULAR FITNESS (MUSCLE STRENGTH AND MUSCLE ENDURANCE)

Why Evaluate the Muscular Fitness of People With DCD?

A description of muscular fitness (muscle strength and muscle endurance) and its relevance to health in general is provided in Chapter 2, and as with cardiorespiratory fitness, this information would also apply to people with DCD. For example, poorer muscular fitness in children is associated with an increased risk profile for future cardiovascular diseases (García-Hermoso et al. 2019).

In addition, children with DCD have reduced muscle strength and endurance compared to their typically developing peers (Rivilis et al. 2011) and people with DCD do not show increases in muscle strength at the same rate as their typically developing peers with growth (Demers et al. 2020). These deficits may explain in part the increased cardiovascular risk seen in people with DCD (Joshi et al. 2015). Thus, similar to cardiorespiratory fitness, an evaluation of muscular fitness might provide valuable information to people with DCD, their families, clinicians, physical activity professionals, or researchers regarding whether or not it is low and consequently whether or not it might be beneficial to improve it to help decrease risks for poor heart health over time. Repeating a given test can be used to determine changes over time or after an intervention.

How to Evaluate the Muscular Fitness of People With DCD

LABORATORY TESTS

Muscle strength can be measured with an isokinetic dynamometer with people with DCD (Raynor 2001). Using such a device means muscle strength can be assessed throughout the range of motion at a pre-set, constant speed (Baltzopoulos and Kellis 1998). When testing with an isokinetic dynamometer, the limb is supported by an attachment, and children may need a particularly small attachment given the size of their limbs compared to those of an adult (Gaul 1995). A practice session is often recommended so the individual learns what is required of them (Baltzopoulos and Kellis 1998) and two to four trials are needed to obtain a maximal result (Gaul 1995). **Muscle endurance** can be measured in people with DCD using the Wingate Anaerobic test as described in Chapter 2. Children with DCD as young as 4 years old can successfully complete the Wingate Anaerobic test (King-Dowling et al. 2018). See King-Dowling et al. (2018) for the specific protocol for this group. Note that individuals with more severe motor delays or muscular weakness may require a reduction (75%) of the typical load (O'Beirne et al. 1994).

FIELD TESTS OF MUSCLE STRENGTH (INDIVIDUAL MUSCLE GROUPS)

Maximal isometric muscle strength (defined in Chapter 2) of individual muscle groups of the arms and legs (with the exception of the calf muscles) can be measured with a hand-held dynamometer if the evaluator (often a physical therapist) has the necessary skills (specialized training and recent experience). See Hebert et al. (2015) for directions for using a hand-held dynamometer. These directions have been used to evaluate the strength of the leg muscles of children with DCD (Demers et al. 2020). There is no known reason why the strength of the arm muscles could not also be evaluated with these directions. The link also provides results from this hand-held dynamometer test for a large group of typically developing children aged 4 to 17 years old. Values for a child or adolescent with DCD can be compared to the reference values for their age and sex to help determine if weakness exists. **Calf muscle strength** can be estimated using the unilateral heel rise test (Yocum et al. 2010). Briefly, the person stands facing a wall, using their fingertips to support themselves minimally against the wall. The non-tested leg is then bent up so the foot is off the floor. A maximum heel rise (rising up on toes) with the other leg (the tested leg) is done. The evaluator points a laser on the wall for a target (50% of the vertical distance of the maximum heel rise). The individual being evaluated performs as many heel rises as they can at a pace of 2 seconds per rise, and they need to make the laser on the wall disappear each time. The test ends if two heel rises in a row are not successful. This means the pace is not kept up, the height is not sufficient (laser target does not disappear), the other foot touches the floor, or the individual bends forward on the wall (supporting with more than their fingertips). The score is the number of successful heel rises. The test can be repeated to determine change over time or following an intervention.

FIELD TESTS OF GLOBAL LEG MUSCLE STRENGTH

Should the intent be to estimate leg muscle strength globally (as might be done when screening for muscle weakness), the standing long jump (also known as the standing broad jump) can be used (Fernandez-Santos et al. 2015), including for children as young as 4 years old with DCD (King-Dowling et al. 2017; Bulten et al. 2019). For this test, children are required to stand with both feet behind a marked line and jump as far forward as they can using a two-footed take-off and landing. Usually two to three trials are performed, with the best jump recorded. Distance measured is taken from the line to the back of the closest heel. Children with DCD may require additional demonstration and instruction due to difficulties landing or taking off on two feet. See De Miguel-Etayo et al. (2014) for the reference values in percentiles for typically developing males and females aged 6 to 9 years old. See Ortega et al. (2011) for similar reference values but for young people aged 13 to 17 years old. These values can be used to determine if the child or young person has reduced strength globally in the muscles of the legs. As with the percentile values for the 20m shuttle run test, a percentile of 50 for a given child would mean 50% of children or young people of the same age and sex have a global leg strength value below the child or young person's value.

Field test of muscle endurance can be estimated in those with DCD using the Muscle Power Sprint Test (Aertssen et al. 2016). This test requires children to perform six 15m sprints, with a 10-second rest between each sprint. See Verschuren et al. (2007) for the directions for the test (originally developed for children with CP). See Douma-van Riet et al. (2012) for the results from this test for a large group of typically developing 6 to 12-year-old children. One can compare the results of a given child with DCD in this age range to their typically developing peers of the same height and sex to determine if low muscle endurance exists and, if so, its extent.

DCD-Specific Training Principles for Muscular Fitness

As with cardiorespiratory fitness, training targeting muscular fitness can be done as part of healthy lifestyle or, should it be low, to reduce the risk for poor cardiovascular health over time (García-Hermoso et al. 2019).

MUSCLE STRENGTH-SPECIFIC TRAINING PRINCIPLES

The muscle strength training principles for children and adults as covered in Chapter 2 also apply to individuals with DCD. As with cardiorespiratory fitness training, what is most important for the individual with DCD who wishes to improve muscle strength is that the training program is safe and that it can be done over the long-term. Thus, the training program and its context need to be acceptable, feasible, and interesting for the individual. The program should be supervised to ensure the training is performed correctly for optimum results and to avoid injury. Adults or older adolescents with DCD who have experience with strength training may wish to consult a professional and determine with them the level of supervision that is needed. See Kordi et al. (2016) for a specific training program that has been associated with an improvement in muscle strength in children with DCD.

MUSCLE ENDURANCE-SPECIFIC TRAINING PRINCIPLES

In general, the principles as laid out in Chapter 2 apply to those with DCD. However, very little is known about the effects of only muscle endurance training in DCD.

BODY COMPOSITION

Why Evaluate the Body Composition of People With DCD?

Body composition, especially body fat (body adiposity) and its importance for health, including heart health, are reviewed in general in Chapter 2; this importance is also true for those with DCD. Moreover, children with DCD appear to have an increased risk for being overweight or obese (Hendrix et al. 2014). This risk may increase with age and the extent of the movement difficulties; it is also greater in males compared to females (Hendrix et al. 2014). Finally, people with DCD are at an increased risk for diseases related to obesity (Joshi et al. 2015).

Thus, similar to cardiorespiratory and muscular fitness, an evaluation of body composition can provide valuable information to people with DCD, their families, clinicians, physical activity professionals, or researchers regarding whether or not the individual with DCD is overweight or obese. Finally, should it be decided that an intervention to improve body composition is required, the body size and composition measurements can be taken again after the intervention to determine its effect.

How to Evaluate the Body Composition of People With DCD

LABORATORY TESTS

The criterion standard, dual-energy X-ray absorptiometry (described in Chapter 2), has been used for those with DCD (Yam and Fong 2018). In addition, bioelectric impedance analysis (also described in Chapter 2) can be used to assess body fat percentage in children with DCD (King-Dowling et al. 2018).

FIELD TESTS

In addition to standard height and weight measurements to determine body mass index (see Chapter 2 for details), waist circumference is a simple measure that has been used for people with DCD (Hendrix et al. 2014). Cut-points specific to DCD for determining overweight and obese status do not yet exist so one can use values from the general population for an estimate. For children, one can use the following charts to determine what centile the waist circumference is closest to given the child's age and sex (https://cpeg-gcep.net/sites/default/files/upload/bookfiles/WC_M_Dec2015.pdf and https://cpeg-gcep.net/sites/default/files/upload/bookfiles/WC_F_Dec2015.pdf). As with other reference values organized as centiles, a centile of 50 for a specific child would mean 50% of children have a waist circumference below the child's value. A child could be considered obese if their waist circumference is at or above the 93rd centile for their age and sex (Sharma et al. 2015). They could be considered overweight if it is at or above the 75th centile (but not at or above the 93rd) (Sharma et al. 2015).

For adults, the criterion is waist circumference itself (Ross et al. 2020). Obesity is defined as a waist circumference of ≥105cm for females and ≥110cm for males. Overweight for females is defined as ≥90cm (except if ≥105cm) and for males it is ≥100cm (except if ≥110 cm).

Effects of Physical Activity on the Body Composition of People With DCD

Little is known about the effects of physical activity on body composition in children or adults with DCD. What is recommended to address overweight and obesity for children with physical disabilities is a holistic approach that considers physical activity and nutrition (McPherson et al. 2016). Thus, people with DCD who wish to address body composition issues may wish to consult with professionals in both physical activity and nutrition with experience with this group.

FLEXIBILITY

Why Evaluate the Flexibility of People With DCD?

Flexibility and its importance to general function are reviewed in Chapter 2. For people with DCD, there is a great deal of individual variability in their flexibility with some children showing reduced flexibility and some showing increased flexibility (Hands and Larkin 2002). Among those showing increased flexibility, some may be similar to people with joint hypermobility syndrome (e.g. show joint pain, flat feet) (Kirby and Davies 2007).

Since both too much and too little flexibility may contribute to injury during physical activities, those wishing to increase their level of physical activity or engage activities with quick and brisk movements should consult a health care professional with experience with DCD and such issues.

How to Evaluate the Flexibility of People With DCD

Laboratory Tests

Laboratory tests are not typically used for measuring flexibility in this population.

Field Test of Flexibility (Individual Muscle Groups)

A **goniometer or an inclinometer** as described in Chapter 2 and detailed in Chapter 6 can be used. This is typically done by a health care professional such as a physical therapist when the flexibility of specific muscles groups is of interest, perhaps as related to participation in a specific sport or following a sports injury.

Field Tests of the Flexibility of Back Muscles and Muscles That Straighten the Hips and Knees

The most commonly used test of this type for people with DCD (Rivilis et al. 2011) is the **sit and reach test** (American College of Sports Medicine 2013). This test measures the flexibility of the lower back muscles and the muscles behind the hips and knees (those that straighten the hips and knees). The test might be done when screening for back and leg flexibility issues. To perform this test, the individual sits on the floor with their knees straight and places the soles of their feet against the edge of a bench or box. Then, placing one hand directly on top of the other, they reach forward as far as they can without bending their knees. The most distant point that they are able to reach along the top of the bench or box is measured. With the **back-saver version of the test** (Ortega et al. 2011; De Miguel-Etayo et al. 2014), the flexibility of the back muscles along with the muscles behind the hip and knee of each side are measured separately. This means rather than having the soles of both feet against the box, only the sole of one foot is. The other leg (non-measured leg) is bent at the hip and knee so that the foot is flat on the ground. See De Miguel-Etayo et al. (2014) for the reference values in percentiles for typically developing males and females 6 to 9 years old. See Ortega et al. (2011) for similar reference values, but for young people 13 to 17 years old. These values are for the back-saver version of the test, and they can be used to determine if the child or young person has reduced flexibility of back muscles and the muscles that straighten the hips and knees of one leg or the other. As with the percentile values for the 20m shuttle run test and the standing long jump test, a percentile of 50 for a given child would mean 50% of children or young people of the same age and sex have a flexibility value below the child or young person's value.

Effects of Physical Activity on the Flexibility of People With DCD

The impact of physical activity on flexibility has not been specifically studied with people with DCD. General recommendations for flexibility exercises are mentioned in Chapter 2 and would hold true for people with DCD, unless specific flexibility issues (increased or decreased) have been identified for a given individual by a professional such as a physical therapist. In this case the individual would follow the recommendations of the professional.

PROMOTING A PHYSICALLY ACTIVE LIFESTYLE FOR PEOPLE WITH DCD

The physical and mental health benefits of physical activity for the general population are well known (Janssen and Leblanc 2010) and detailed in Chapter 2. This information applies to people with DCD. How to assess physical activity is discussed in Chapter 4 and general information on how to promote a physically active lifestyle across the lifespan can be found in Chapter 5. This information also applies to people with DCD. The following paragraphs provide DCD-specific information on promoting a physically active lifestyle.

One major concern regarding children with DCD is that their lower levels of physical activity, relative to typically developing children (Cairney et al. 2010b), may mean they will not experience the optimal benefits of a healthy active lifestyle. Children with DCD may be less active due to a variety of physical and psychosocial factors in addition to their motor challenges including lower fitness (Rivilis et al. 2011), lower self-confidence (Cairney et al. 2005), and less enjoyment in physical activities (Cairney et al. 2007). This is of particular concern as both physical inactivity in childhood have been shown to track into adolescence and at least into early adulthood (Janz et al. 2000). In other words, the (in)activity profiles of children with DCD may persist into the future unless specific strategies are put in place to foster increased physical activity.

Recently, recommendations to foster participation in physical activities of children with DCD have been developed in a guide (Demers et al. 2022). The 30 points in the guide were established after an extensive review of current scientific evidence and current practices. The guide was formulated in consultation with parents, educators, and physical activity leaders in the community as well with as clinicians. There are specific sections to address the role of each of these groups in supporting the child with DCD in their participation in physical activities for the following areas: (1) choice of activity or activities; (2) how to help ensure the choice is in keeping with the child's interests and abilities; and (3) how to help the child learn new movements prior to engaging in the activity if and when necessary. The child is at the heart of all recommendations. Adults with DCD can also use the guide as a starting point.

Here are a few key points from the guide:

1. The ideal activity will be that which appeals to the child's interests and abilities and can be done safely.
2. Input from the child's rehabilitation professional or physical education teacher can be helpful in better understanding the child's abilities.
3. Pictures of activities can be used to help understand the child's interests.
4. The child's efforts should be highlighted and rewarded with an emphasis on participation in and enjoyment of the activity rather than on the level of performance.
5. When the child is learning new skills, they should be encouraged to: (1) determine what they want to achieve (goal); (2) develop their plan to achieve the goal; (3) check whether they have achieved the goal; and (4) modify the plan as needed. Parents, educators, physical activity leaders in the community, and clinicians can help the child with each of these steps as needed.

REFERENCES

Aertssen WFM, Ferguson GD, Smits-Engelsman BCM (2016) Performance on Functional Strength Measurement and Muscle Power Sprint Test confirm poor anaerobic capacity in children with Developmental Coordination Disorder. *Res Dev Disabil* **59**: 115–126.

American College of Sports Medicine (2013) *ACSM's Guidelines for Exercise Testing and Prescription.* Baltimore, MD: Lippincott Williams & Wilkins.

American Psychiatric Association (2013) *Diagnostic and Statistical Manual of Mental Disorders, Fifth Edition (DSM V).* Arlington, VA: American Psychiatric Association.

Baltzopoulos V, Kellis E (1998) Isokinetic strength during childhood and adolescence. In: Van Praagh E, editor, *Pediatric Anaerobic Performance.* Champaign, IL: Human Kinetics, pp 225–240.

Blank R, Barnett AL, Cairney J et al. (2019) International clinical practice recommendations on the definition, diagnosis, assessment, intervention, and psychosocial aspects of developmental coordination disorder. *Dev Med Child Neurol* **61**: 242–285.

Buckley J, Cohen JD, Kramer AF, McAuley E, Mullen SP (2014) Cognitive control in the self-regulation of physical activity and sedentary behavior. *Frontiers in Human Neuroscience* **8**: 747.

Bulten R, King-Dowling S, Cairney J (2019) Assessing the validity of standing long jump to predict muscle power in children with and without motor delays. *Pediatric Exercise Science* **31**: 432–437.

Cacau LA, De Santana-Filho VJ, Maynard LG, Gomes MN, Fernandes M, Carvalho VO (2016) Reference values for the six-minute walk test in healthy children and adolescents: a systematic review. *Braz J Cardiovasc Surg* **31**: 381–388.

Cairney J, Hay JA, Faught BE, Wade TJ, Corna L, Flouris A (2005) Developmental coordination disorder, generalized self-efficacy toward physical activity, and participation in organized and free play activities. *J Pediatr* **147**: 515–520.

Cairney J, Hay J, Mandigo J, Wade T, Faught BE, Flouris A (2007) Developmental coordination disorder and reported enjoyment of physical education in children. *European Physical Education Review* **13**: 81–98.

Cairney J, Hay J, Veldhuizen S, Faught B (2010a) Comparison of VO2 maximum obtained from 20m shuttle run and cycle ergometer in children with and without developmental coordination disorder. *Res Dev Disabil* **31**: 1332–1339.

Cairney J, Hay JA, Veldhuizen S, Missiuna C, Faught BE (2010b) Developmental coordination disorder, sex, and activity deficit over time: a longitudinal analysis of participation trajectories in children with and without coordination difficulties. *Dev Med Child Neurol* **52**: e67–72.

Cairney J, King-Dowling S (2015) Developmental Coordination Disorder. In: Matson JL, editor, *Comorbid Conditions Among Children with Autism Spectrum Disorders*. Switzerland: Springer International Publishing, pp 303–322.

Camden C, Wilson B, Kirby A, Sugden D, Missiuna C (2015) Best practice principles for management of children with developmental coordination disorder (DCD): results of a scoping review. *Child: Care, Health and Development* **41**: 147–159.

De Miguel-Etayo P, Gracia-Marco L, Ortega FB et al. (2014) Physical fitness reference standards in European children: the IDEFICS study. *Int J Obes (Lond)* **38**: S57–S66. **https://www.nature.com/articles/ijo2014136.pdf**.

Demers I, Corriveau G, Morneau-Vaillancourt G et al. (2022) A clinical practice guide to enhance physical activity participation for children with developmental coordination disorder in Canada. *Physiother Can.* (aop), p.e20210071.

Demers I, Moffet H, Hebert L, Maltais DB (2020) Growth and muscle strength development in children with developmental coordination disorder. *Dev Med Child Neurol* **62**: 1082–1088.

Douma-Van Riet D, Verschuren O, Jelsma D, Kruitwagen C, Smits-Engelsman B, Takken T (2012) Reference values for the muscle power sprint test in 6- to 12-year-old children. *Pediatr Phys Ther* **24**: 327–332. **https://journals.lww.com/pedpt/Fulltext/2012/24040/Reference_Values_for_the_Muscle_Power_Sprint_Test.7.aspx**.

Farhat F, Masmoudi K, Hsairi I et al. (2015) The effects of 8 weeks of motor skill training on cardio-respiratory fitness and endurance performance in children with developmental coordination disorder. *Applied Physiology, Nutrition, and Metabolism* **40**: 1269–1278.

Fernandez-Santos JR, Ruiz JR, Cohen DD, Gonzalez-Montesinos JL, Castro-Piñero J (2015) Reliability and validity of tests to assess lower-body muscular power in children. *The Journal of Strength & Conditioning Research* **29**: 2277–2285.

García-Hermoso A, Ramírez-Campillo R, Izquierdo M (2019) Is muscular fitness associated with future health benefits in children and adolescents? A systematic review and meta-analysis of longitudinal studies. *Sports Medicine* **49**: 1079–1094.

Gaul CA (1995) Muscular strength and endurance. In: Docherty D, editor, *Measurement in Pediatric Exercise Science*. Champaign, IL: Human Kinetics, pp 225–254.

Geuze RH (2005) Postural control in children with developmental coordination disorder. *Neural Plast* **12**: 183–196; discussion 263–272.

Gibbs J, Appleton J, Appleton R (2007) Dyspraxia or developmental coordination disorder? Unravelling the enigma. *Archives of Disease in Childhood* **92**: 534–539.

Gubbay S, Ellis E, Walton J (1975) *Clumsy Children: A Study of Developmental Apraxic and Agnostic Ataxia*. London: W. Saunders.

Hands B, Larkin D (2002) Physical fitness and developmental coordination disorder. In: Cermak S, Larkin D, editors, *Developmental Coordination Disorder*. Albany, NY: Delmar, pp 174–184.

Hebert LJ, Maltais DB, Lepage C, Saulnier J, Crete M (2015) Hand-held dynamometry isometric torque reference values for children and adolescents. *Pediatr Phys Ther* **27**: 414–423. **https://www.ncbi.nlm.nih.gov/pmc/articles/PMC4581449/pdf/ppyty-27-414.pdf**.

Henderson SE, Henderson L (2003) Toward an understanding of developmental coordination disorder: terminological and diagnostic issues. *Neural Plasticity* **10**: 1–13.

Henderson S, Sugden D (2007) *The Movement Assessment Battery for Children*, 2nd ed. London: Pearson Assessment.

Hendrix CG, Prins MR, Dekkers H (2014) Developmental coordination disorder and overweight and obesity in children: a systematic review. *Obes Rev* **15**: 408–423.

Henriksson H, Henriksson P, Tynelius P et al. (2020) Cardiorespiratory fitness, muscular strength, and obesity in adolescence and later chronic disability due to cardiovascular disease: a cohort study of 1 million men. *European Heart Journal* **41**: 1503–1510.

Hofmann W, Schmeichel BJ, Baddeley AD (2012) Executive functions and self-regulation. *Trends in Cognitive Sciences* **16**: 174–180.

Holsti L, Grunau RV, Whitfield MF (2002) Developmental coordination disorder in extremely low birth weight children at nine years. *Journal of Developmental & Behavioral Pediatrics* **23**: 9–15.

Janssen I, Leblanc AG (2010) Systematic review of the health benefits of physical activity and fitness in school-aged children and youth. *Int J Behav Nutr Phys Act* **7**: 40.

Janz KF, Dawson JD, Mahoney LT (2000) Tracking physical fitness and physical activity from childhood to adolescence: the muscatine study. *Med Sci Sports Exerc* **32**: 1250–1257.

Joshi D, Missiuna C, Hanna S, Hay J, Faught BE, Cairney J (2015) Relationship between BMI, waist circumference, physical activity and probable developmental coordination disorder over time. *Hum Mov Sci* **40**: 237–247.

King-Dowling S, Proudfoot NA, Cairney J, Timmons BW (2017) Validity of field assessments to predict peak muscle power in preschoolers. *Applied Physiology, Nutrition, and Metabolism* **42**: 850–854.

King-Dowling S, Rodriguez C, Missiuna C, Timmons BW, Cairney J (2018) Health-related fitness in preschool children with and without motor delays. *Med Sci Sports Exerc* **50**: 1442–1448. **https://journals.lww.com/acsm-msse/Fulltext/2018/07000/Health_related_Fitness_in_Preschool_Children_with.12.aspx**.

Kirby A, Davies R (2007) Developmental Coordination Disorder and Joint Hypermobility Syndrome: overlapping disorders? Implications for research and clinical practice. *Child Care Health Dev* **33**: 513–519.

Kordi H, Sohrabi M, Saberi Kakhki A, Attarzadeh Hossini SR (2016) The effect of strength training based on process approach intervention on balance of children with developmental coordination disorder. *Arch Argent Pediatr* **114**: 526–533. **https://www.sap.org.ar/docs/publicaciones/archivosarg/2016/v114n6a09e.pdf**.

Li AM, Yin J, Au JT et al. (2007) Standard reference for the six-minute-walk test in healthy children aged 7 to 16 years. *Am J Respir Crit Care Med* **176**: 174–180. **https://www.atsjournals.org/doi/pdf/10.1164/rccm.200607-883OC**.

McPherson AC, Ball GD, Maltais DB et al. (2016) A call to action: setting the research agenda for addressing obesity and weight-related topics in children with physical disabilities. *Child Obes* **12**: 59–69.

Mischel W, Ayduk O, Berman MG et al. (2011) 'Willpower' over the life span: decomposing self-regulation. *Social Cognitive and Affective Neuroscience* **6**: 252–256.

Miyake A, Friedman NP, Emerson MJ, Witzki AH, Howerter A, Wager TD (2000) The unity and diversity of executive functions and their contributions to complex 'frontal lobe' tasks: a latent variable analysis. *Cogn Psychol* **41**: 49–100.

O'Beirne C, Larkin D, Cable T (1994) Coordination problems and anaerobic performance in children. *Adapted Physical Activity Quarterly* **11**: 141–149.

Ortega FB, Artero EG, Ruiz JR et al. (2011) Physical fitness levels among European adolescents: the HELENA study. *Br J Sports Med* **45**: 20–29. **http://helenastudy.com/files/Ortega-BJSM-2011.pdf**.

Pujalte GG, Maynard JR, Thurston MJ, Taylor III WC, Chauhan M (2019) Considerations in the care of athletes with attention deficit hyperactivity disorder. *Clinical Journal of Sport Medicine* **29**: 245–256.

Raynor AJ (2001) Strength, power, and coactivation in children with developmental coordination disorder. *Dev Med Child Neurol* **43**: 676–684.

Rivilis I, Hay J, Cairney J, Kleroi P, Liu J, Faught BE (2011) Physical activity and fitness in children with developmental coordination disorder: a systematic review. *Res Dev Disabil* **32**: 894–910.

Ross R, Neeland IJ, Yamashita S et al. (2020) Waist circumference as a vital sign in clinical practice: a consensus statement from the IAS and ICCR Working Group on visceral obesity. *Nat Rev Endocrinol* **16**: 177–189.

Ruiz JR, Castro-Pinero J, Artero EG et al. (2009) Predictive validity of health-related fitness in youth: a systematic review. *Br J Sports Med* **43**: 909–923.

Sharma AK, Metzger DL, Daymont C, Hadjiyannakis S, Rodd CJ (2015) LMS tables for waist-circumference and waist-height ratio Z-scores in children aged 5–19 y in NHANES III: association with cardio-metabolic risks. *Pediatr Res* **78**: 723–729.

Smits-Engelsman BC, Blank R, Van der Kaay AC et al. (2013) Efficacy of interventions to improve motor performance in children with developmental coordination disorder: a combined systematic review and meta-analysis. *Dev Med Child Neurol* **55**: 229–237.

Sugden DA, Chambers ME (2003) Intervention in children with developmental coordination disorder: the role of parents and teachers. *British Journal of Educational Psychology* **73**: 545–561.

Sugden D, Chambers M, Utley A (2006) *Leeds Consensus Statement: Developmental Coordination Disorder as a Specific Learning Difficulty*. Leeds: DCD-UK/Dyscovery Centre.

Verschuren O, Takken T, Ketelaar M, Gorter JW, Helders PJ (2007) Reliability for running tests for measuring agility and anaerobic muscle power in children and adolescents with cerebral palsy. *Pediatr Phys Ther* **19**: 108–115. **https://journals.lww.com/pedpt/Fulltext/2007/01920/Reliability_for_Running_Tests_for_Measuring.2.aspx**.

Wilson PH, Maruff P, Ives S, Currie J (2001) Abnormalities of motor and praxis imagery in children with DCD. *Human Movement Science* **20**: 135–159.

Wilson PH, McKenzie BE (1998) Information processing deficits associated with developmental coordination disorder: a meta-analysis of research findings. *The Journal of Child Psychology and Psychiatry and Allied Disciplines* **39**: 829–840.

Wilson PH, Smits-Engelsman B, Caeyenberghs K et al. (2017) Cognitive and neuroimaging findings in developmental coordination disorder: new insights from a systematic review of recent research. *Developmental Medicine & Child Neurology* **59**: 1117–1129.

Wilson PH, Thomas PR, Maruff P (2002) Motor imagery training ameliorates motor clumsiness in children. *Journal of Child Neurology* **17**: 491–498.

Wright HC, Sugden DA (1996) The nature of developmental coordination disorder: inter-and intragroup differences. *Adapted Physical Activity Quarterly* **13**: 357–371.

Yam TTT, Fong SSM (2018) Leg muscle activation patterns during walking and leg lean mass are different in children with and without developmental coordination disorder. *Res Dev Disabil* **73**: 87–95.

Yocum A, McCoy SW, Bjornson KF, Mullens P, Burton GN (2010) Reliability and validity of the standing heel-rise test. *Phys Occup Ther Pediatr* **30**: 190–204.

Zwicker JG, Missiuna C, Boyd LA (2009) Neural correlates of developmental coordination disorder: a review of hypotheses. *Journal of Child Neurology* **24**: 1273–1281.

Zwicker JG, Missiuna C, Harris SR, Boyd LA (2012) Developmental coordination disorder: a review and update. *European Journal of Paediatric Neurology* **16**: 573–581.

CHAPTER 8

Spina Bifida and Childhood-Acquired Spinal Cord Injury

Ana-Marie Rojas and Shubhra Mukherjee

The chapter begins with an overview of spina bifida (including common impairments, comorbidities, and medications. This is followed by an overview of childhood-acquired spinal cord injury (SCI) using the same structure. Next, components of health-related fitness that are covered in this book (cardiorespiratory fitness and submaximal exercise capacity, muscular fitness, body composition, flexibility) are discussed (see Chapter 2 for definitions of these terms). For each component, the reasons why it might be evaluated are noted, followed by information on how to evaluate it and finally by either training principles specific to spina bifida and childhood-acquired SCI (cardiorespiratory fitness, muscular fitness) or how physical activity affects the component (body composition, flexibility). The chapter concludes with suggestions for promoting a physically active lifestyle for people with spina bifida or childhood-acquired SCI.

Note that the tests used to evaluate the various health-related fitness components are classed as laboratory or field tests. As mentioned in Chapter 2, laboratory tests are typically used in research or specialized clinical settings, whereas field tests can be used in research, clinical, and community settings.

Throughout the chapter, when the reader is referred to resources by the statement 'see Author et al. (year)' or when article URLs are mentioned in the table legends, that means the article or document cited is freely available on the internet and the URL or other information needed to locate the article or document is found following the corresponding reference in the reference list.

WHAT IS SPINA BIFIDA?

Spina bifida refers to structural changes affecting the spinal cord and some parts of the brain that are present at birth. These changes are due to incomplete closure of the neural tube, the hollow structure from which the brain and spina cord will develop in utero (before birth). Spina bifida is part of a broader classification of neural tube defects (NTDs), which are the second most prevalent defects present at birth worldwide. NTDs can be classified as open or closed based on whether or not the neural tissue is exposed. Open NTDs involve both spinal cord and brainstem. Closed NTDs are usually confined to the spine. Spina bifida, also known as myelomeningocele, is the most common NTD. Spina bifida can be classified by location: cervical (spine at the neck), thoracic (spine at the upper back), lumbar (spine at the lower back), and sacral (lowest part of the spine). The closer to the head the NDT is located, the more severe the impairments, associated conditions, and complications will likely be.

The national Spina Bifida Association documents more than 70 000 individuals in the United States living with spina bifida and estimates true numbers to be over twice that. Each year 1500 babies are born with spina bifida (Parker et al. 2010). Individuals with spina bifida will likely require surgical procedures early in life (Adzick et al. 2011). Neural tube closure can be performed in utero (before birth) or should be surgically done within 48 to 72 hours after birth for best outcomes and reduced risk of infection.

COMMON IMPAIRMENTS AND COMORBIDITIES WITH SPINA BIFIDA

People with spina bifida frequently have associated impairments and comorbidities. Those that could affect safely engaging in physical activity are described below, including common signs and symptoms, medical treatment, and any safety considerations related to physical activity. For an individual with spina bifida who has one or more of these impairments or comorbidities, it is prudent to seek medical clearance before they begin a new programme of physical activity, especially if they have not been physically active in the past.

Hydrocephalus

Hydrocephalus, an increase in cerebrospinal fluid in cavities (ventricles) that are found deep in the brain, occurs in the majority of children with spina bifida. It is due to an obstruction of the flow of cerebrospinal fluid and it results in increased pressure in the brain. A ventricular shunt is introduced in order to relieve pressure in the brain by redirecting the fluid into another cavity such as the abdominal cavity. However, sometimes the shunt may stop providing adequate pressure relief, possibly due to an infection, an obstruction, or a valve or catheter (tube) malfunction (Hampton et al. 2011). In children and adults, symptoms of high pressure in the brain can be subtle or intermittent, with headache, vomiting, lethargy, reduced cognitive or school function, or brainstem symptoms such as swallowing issues. In severe situations, heart rate and breathing may be compromised, and associated compression and herniation of brain structures may occur. It is important that the family, the person themselves, and all individuals who supervise physical activity programmes are aware of these signs and symptoms and that the individual with spina bifida be brought to immediate medical attention if they arise. Failure to do so can be life-threatening.

Chiari II Malformation

Chiari II malformation is the most common hindbrain abnormality in spina bifida. It is characterized by compression and protrusion of the back parts of the brain through the opening in the skull for the spinal cord (Juranek et al. 2010). People with a Chiari II malformation may also have hydrocephalus, facial paralysis, swallowing and nasal difficulties, altered mental status, sleep apnoea (where breathing during sleep breathing repeatedly stops and starts), arm weakness, and changes in muscle tone (underlying stiffness in muscles) (Adzick 2012). Symptoms may be severe and require immediate surgical treatment. In severe cases, the need for mechanical help for breathing may result. Clearance for physical activity should be obtained from the neurosurgeon. Any decline in cognitive function should be met with caution and evaluated medically. See also Chapter 10 for details on adaptions to testing and programming for people with reduced cognitive function.

Tethering of the Spinal Cord and Other Spinal Cord Changes

Tethering of the spinal cord is a condition where there is traction of the spinal cord because the spinal nerves have become bound to the scarring in and around the site of closure of the NTD and the spinal cord is less able to grow as the child grows. Loss or changes in sensation in legs, changes in motor ability or strength, increased tone or spasticity (a type of increased muscle stiffness), rapid progression of scoliosis (curvature of the spine), back and leg pain, and changes in bladder function are some signs and symptoms that may indicate tethered cord syndrome. Another spinal cord change (pathology) that may be seen in spina bifida is the development of syrinx or enlarged fluid cavities in the spinal cord. Symptoms can be similar to those found with a tethered cord. Although not as an immediate, possibly life-threatening situation as increased pressure in the brain, it is still important that the family, the person themselves, and all individuals who supervise physical training or exercise programmes be aware of the signs and symptoms of a tethered cord and syrinx and that the individual's physician be informed as soon as possible if these signs and symptoms arise. In the case of a suspected tethered cord, surgery may be necessary in some cases to de-tether the spinal cord especially if recent or progressive functional loss is noted.

Neurogenic Bowel and Neurogenic Bladder

Neurogenic bowel and neurogenic bladder are conditions of bowl and bladder dysfunction that occur when there is no longer sufficient communication between the brain and the nerves in the spinal cord that control bladder and bowel function. In the case of people with spina bifida, the lack of communication between the brain and these nerves is because of the spinal NTD. People with neurogenic bowel and neurogenic bladder may have a loss of bowel and bladder control and increased frequency in the need to empty the bowel and bladder. People with a neurogenic bowel may also have constipation or even a lack of bowel movements. People with a neurogenic bladder may be unable to empty the bladder and thus they may have an increased risk for urinary tract infections (UTIs). Problems related to neurogenic bowel or neurogenic bladder often require medical management and possible surgical intervention (Leibold et al. 2000; Bauer 2003; Cardona-Grau and Chiang 2017). Optimal medical management can help regulate function and reduce or avoid incontinence.

A UTI is of particular concern, as it is the most frequent cause of hospitalizations in people with spina bifida. Furthermore, signs and symptoms of UTI may also be atypical for people with spina bifida because of sensory deficits, but they often include one or more of the following: abdominal discomfort or pressure, leaking or episodes of incontinence, malodorous urine, increased urinary frequency, fever, fatigue, and altered mental status. To help maintain bladder continence and health, intermittent bladder self-catheterization may be required. This is where a catheter (tube) is used to drain urine at regular intervals during the day. When the person is unable to access the tube that allows urine to pass out of the body (in the penis in males and just above the vagina in females), surgery may to needed to create an opening between the bladder and the belly button to facilitate catheterizing techniques to empty the bladder.

For bowel care, surgery may also be needed to provide a catheterizable opening through the abdominal wall to flush the large intestine from the proximal end with an enema (Perez et al. 2001).

Medications used for bowel and bladder management may affect the function of the nerves that control the bowl and bladder, and pre-existing bowel and bladder issues may be exacerbated during physical activity. Emptying the bladder and bowel is therefore recommended prior to physical activity to prevent leakage and other issues.

The family, the person themselves, and all individuals who supervise physical training or exercise programmes must therefore be aware of the signs and symptoms of neurogenic bowel and neurogenic bladder and of a UTI as well as the importance of emptying the bowel and bladder before physical activity. In the case of a UTI (or really any unexplained change in bladder or bowel function), the person should be referred to their physician so it can be assessed and treated as soon as possible.

Autonomic Dysfunction

Autonomic dysfunction is dysfunction of the part of the nervous system that controls the body's automatic responses. Of particular importance to engaging in physical activity is that autonomic dysfunction can result in reduced control of body temperature, which can lead to hyperthermia (abnormal *increase* in core body temperature) or hypothermia (abnormal *decrease* in core body temperature), depending on the situation.

HYPERTHERMIA

Abnormal sweat patterns may reduce the body's ability to dissipate heat (the need of which can increase with physical activity), and if severe, result in heat stroke, which is a severe form of hyperthermia. People with heat stroke can present with slurred speech, confusion, dizziness, hallucinations, syncope (fainting), and muscle cramps. Heat stroke can result in permanent brain damage if severe and is thus an emergency situation where immediate medical assistance much be sought. The person must also be immediately moved to shade or, if possible, to an indoor, air-conditioned space. Excess clothing should be removed and the person should be cooled however possible (e.g. by being moved to a tub of water, given a cool shower, sprayed with a water hose, sponged with cool water with a fan blowing on them, having wet towels placed on their head, neck, armpits, and groin).

Reducing the Risk of Heat Stroke

It is common practice for individuals with neurogenic bladder (see the previous section above for a definition) to limit their fluid intake in order to avoid frequent catheterizations. Failure to anticipate fluid loss through sweating can be a cause of dehydration that, in turn, can also increase the risk for heat stroke. Thus, individuals who are sweating should be encouraged to hydrate even if they are not thirsty and be educated about why this is important even if it leads to more frequent catheterizations. Chapter 3 provides additional information regarding hydration in general during physical activity. In addition to maintaining hydration, the risk of heat stroke during physical activity can be reduced by wearing loose, light coloured clothing that wicks the sweat away and on hot days, avoiding the sun between 11am and 3pm.

HYPOTHERMIA

Poor temperature regulation can also result in hypothermia if the individual is engaging in physical activity in cold, rainy, and windy weather. People with hypothermia can present with confusion, drowsiness, a reduced heart rate, and uncontrolled shivering and weakness. If the person is showing the signs and symptoms of hypothermia, they should be moved to a warm, dry environment and medical attention sought if the signs and symptoms continue after they are moved.

Reducing the Risk of Hypothermia

Prevention of loss of body heat by wearing appropriate dry clothing or clothing that maintains heat when wet can be helpful. It may also be prudent to avoid outside physical activity in particularly cold, rainy, and windy weather, especially if the person has had severe hypothermic episodes in the past.

As with other issues that can arise during physical activity, the family, the individual themselves, and all individuals who supervise physical training or exercise programmes must be aware of the signs and symptoms of heat stroke and hypothermia, what can be done to reduce risks, as well as what to do if these events occur.

Sensory Deficits and Resulting Skin Problems

Sensory deficits increase the risk of pressure ulcers (open sores) and skin breakdown in individuals with spina bifida (Pandey et al. 2015). Wet surfaces, for example due to sweat or a lack of bowel and bladder control (see the above section on neurogenic bowel and neurogenic bladder for details) can also contribute to skin breakdown. Pressure ulcers can be severe enough to require skin grafting or other surgery. If not treated when the open sore first appears, infections can occur that can be life- or limb-threatening, meaning amputation of fingers or toes or even other parts of the arms or legs may have to be performed. For this reason, most people with spina bifida and their families are taught to relieve pressure on the skin by weight shifting every 15 to 20 minutes for 30 seconds or more while sitting or turning every 2 hours while in bed. They are also taught to perform daily visual skin checks of insensate skin areas.

Given that about half of pressure injuries to the skin are equipment-related (Schluer et al. 2009), the equipment used during physical activities and sports must be evaluated to ensure proper fit as well as sufficient cushioning and pressure distribution before a new physical activity programme is begun. This should be done by a person knowledgeable in the proper fit of the equipment, such as a clinician or technician. People with spina bifida who undergo changes in body composition (see Chapter 2 for a definition) or growth or any other changes to their body, such as swelling due to extra fluid building up in tissues (lymphedema) that can occur in people with spina bifida (Garcia and Dicianno 2011) are at particular risk for improper equipment fit and therefore skin breakdown. In addition, equipment such as a wheelchair that is left out in the cold or under the sun can reach extreme temperatures and cause a burn to skin with sensory deficits when the individual uses the equipment for their physical activity. Therefore, equipment must be kept in the shade or inside before it is used.

Musculoskeletal Complications

Musculoskeletal complications are frequently seen in people with spina bifida. Muscle imbalance can result in contractures (permanent shortening of muscles and other tissues around a joint that makes the joint stiff and prevents its full movement), scoliosis (spine curvature), and shortening of the limbs or angles at which muscles pull; this in turn can mechanically reduce the force that muscles can produce. To improve mobility and function, individuals with spina bifida may undergo musculoskeletal surgeries or they may use specialized equipment (e.g. leg or trunk braces, wheelchairs, walkers, canes, or crutches) or both. Proper equipment fit is very important to both the intended use of the equipment and to reduce the risk of skin breakdown (see the previous section on sensory deficits and resulting skin problems for details on equipment fitting prior to beginning a new activity programme).

In people who use wheelchairs, overuse injury of the shoulder is common. Inability to propel a wheelchair for people who use them for mobility will have a great impact on an individual's functional mobility and overall independence. Proper wheelchair provision, as well as teaching propulsion techniques and shoulder strengthening, may prevent shoulder injuries (Symonds et al. 2018). Power assist additions may also reduce the stress on the shoulder, as may lightweight equipment that is correctly configured. The reader is also invited to review the section on pain in Chapter 3 for further information pertaining to joint pain.

Finally, people with spina bifida are at an increased risk for fractures, especially if they have decreased bone density or they do not walk a lot. People with spina bifida may not feel or notice a broken bone due to sensory deficits and the only signs of a broken bone may be mild swelling and warmth. A common site for fractures is just above and below the knee, and in some cases the fracture can occur with minimal trauma or twisting movements (Lala et al. 2014). The reader should consult the osteoporosis section in Chapter 3 for further details including what to do to prevent fractures during physical activity. If a fracture is suspected, it is prudent to have this promptly investigated by a physician.

Metabolic Syndrome

People with spinal cord pathology are at an increased risk of obesity and potentially metabolic syndrome (a group of conditions that occur together, increasing risk of heart disease, stroke, and type 2 diabetes); thus exercise and physical activity have special significance. Increasing physical activity is a way to promote health and prevent such complications (Vanhala et al. 1998) as well as potentially improve quality of life. As individuals with spina bifida thrive and seek to achieve their potential, there exists a growing interest in sports and fitness activities.

Hydration and Nutrition Issues

With spina bifida, achieving adequate hydration and nutrition may be challenging, especially if they have difficulty swallowing, which can occur with this condition, or if they have autonomic dysfunction (see the above section on this for a definition) that results in feeling full prematurely. Some people with spina bifida manage their hydration and nutrition with small frequent meals and drinking. If people with spina bifida are having difficulty maintaining hydration and/or nutrition, a tube may be introduced into the stomach to maintain adequate and safe nutrition and/or hydration. In addition, all individuals who supervise physical training or exercise programmes must be aware of the individual's hydration and nutrition issues and how they are managed so they can help support proper management during physical activity. The reader is invited to consult Chapter 3 for general information on hydration and nutrition relevant to physical activity and the previous section on autonomic dysfunction for information on the importance of hydration for body temperature control.

Latex Allergy

Individuals with spina bifida have an increased risk of latex allergy due to frequent exposure since birth (Oomman 2013). Reactions can range from a mild rash or swelling to severe illness including breathing difficulty or airway obstruction and an anaphylactic reaction (a severe life-threatening allergic reaction). Precaution must be taken, and latex products must be avoided, including latex-containing clothing, sports balls, and other handled equipment. See Allergy & Asthma Network (2017) for information about latex free sports equipment.

WHAT IS CHILDHOOD-ACQUIRED SCI?

Childhood-acquired SCI refers to damage to the spinal cord and associate tissues occurring during childhood as the result of trauma, infection, or other (e.g. auto-immune) conditions. Incidence of childhood and adolescent SCI presenting to the emergency department is estimated at 17.5 cases per million or 1308 new cases per year (Selvarajah et al. 2014). Quadriplegia or tetraplegia is a consequence of spinal cord damage resulting in deficits in all four limbs. Paraplegia refers to weakness in the legs, due to a lesion (damage) in the thoracic (mid-back) spinal level or lower. Sometimes the damage to the spinal cord can result in different impairments from one side of the body to the other. SCI is formally classified by the American Spinal Injury Association using the International Standards for Neurological Classification of Spinal Cord Injury. The classification is based upon assessment of strength and sensation at different levels of the body.

Trauma accounts for the majority of cases of SCI. Common causal factors include motor vehicle accidents, falls, violent acts such as gunshot injuries, and sport injuries. Children under the age of 6 years are at higher risk of SCI at the of cervical (neck) level due to their relatively larger head size and relatively weak neck muscles (Bilston and Brown 2007; Selvarajah et al. 2014). SCI without abnormalities visible on X-ray is seen in skeletally immature children. Even though no bone fractures are seen on imaging, injury to the spinal cord may be severe and permanent.

Non-traumatic causes of SCI are uncommon. Transverse myelitis results in cord inflammation and demyelination (damage to the protective coating around nerve fibres). This condition is rare in children but often results in permanent motor and sensory deficits.

Other uncommon but possible causes of childhood-acquired SCI include neoplasms (abnormal tissue growth), compression myelopathy (SCI due to severe compression), toxin (poisons produced by living organisms), infection, or ischemia (reduced oxygen supply due to reduced blood flow) to the spinal cord.

COMMON IMPAIRMENTS AND COMORBIDITIES WITH CHILDHOOD-ACQUIRED SCI

Neurogenic Bowel and Bladder; Autonomic Dysfunction; Sensory Deficits and Resulting Skin Problems; Musculoskeletal Complications; Metabolic Syndrome; Hydration and Nutrition Issues and Latex Allergy

As described above for spina bifida, these impairments can also be seen with people with childhood-acquired SCI. Shortening of the affected arms or legs (noted above), however, is more likely to occur in children who sustain a SCI before the skeleton is mature (while they are still growing). Below are common impairments and comorbidities more commonly seen in SCI.

Autonomic Dysreflexia

A highly dangerous complication of SCI that has occurred above the 6th thoracic level (this is just below shoulder blade level) is autonomic dysreflexia, an overreaction of the involuntary or autonomic nervous system due to stimulation below the level of the SCI (Eldahan and Rabchevsky 2018). Autonomic dysreflexia can result in symptoms such as an increase in blood pressure, sometimes accompanied by a slowing of the heart rate, and it can occur soon after a SCI or much later. In fact, athletes who use a wheelchair have been known to induce autonomic dysreflexia to improve athletic performance (Bhambhani 2002; Mazzeo et al. 2015). Such a 'boosting' practice is dangerous and has been banned in organized athletics for wheelchair users. Other types of stimulation that can lead to autonomic dysreflexia are an over-distended bladder, constipation, ingrown toenails, a fracture, or tissue injury. The symptoms of autonomic dysreflexia can be very severe and even result in death with seizures and swelling of the brain.

The family, the person themselves, and all individuals who supervise physical training or exercise programmes must therefore be aware of the symptoms of autonomic dysreflexia. Should this occur during physical activity, the individual and those supporting them must try to alleviate the issue by having the person sitting upright with their head elevated at 90 degrees until blood pressure reaches a normal level and removing all tight clothing or irritants (such as a full bladder). The person should also seek immediate medical attention as medical management may be required promptly to control blood pressure (Eldahan and Rabchevsky 2018).

Pain and Neuropathic Pain: Increased Tone or Spasticity

These can occur in people with SCI. They are discussed in Chapter 3.

COMMON MEDICATIONS FOR SPINA BIFIDA AND CHILDHOOD-ACQUIRED SCI

People with spina bifida or childhood-acquired SCI are often prescribed long-term medication to help manage some of the complications or associated conditions listed in above sections of this chapter. Some of these medications and their effects on physical activity tolerance are discussed in Chapter 3. However, before new fitness testing and physical activities programmes are undertaken, families of individuals with spina bifida or childhood-acquired SCI who are managing their own health care should speak to their physician about the specific medication the individual is taking and whether the primary or side effects of the medication can affect cardiorespiratory or muscular fitness testing or physical activity tolerance. This information should be shared with all individuals who are supervising and supporting the physical activity of the person with spina bifida or childhood-acquired SCI.

CARDIORESPIRATORY FITNESS AND SUBMAXIMAL EXERCISE CAPACITY

Why Evaluate the Cardiorespiratory Fitness and Submaximal Exercise Capacity of People With Spina Bifida or Childhood-Acquired SCI?

Chapter 2 covers the definitions of cardiorespiratory fitness and submaximal exercise capacity, the difference between children and adults, and why these are important components of health-related fitness. For example, typically developing children who have better cardiorespiratory fitness also have better heart and cardiovascular health as they age (Ruiz et al. 2009; Henriksson et al. 2020). If they improve their cardiorespiratory fitness, they also show an improvement in later heart health (Ruiz et al. 2009). This information would also apply to people with spina bifida or childhood-acquired SCI.

Furthermore, children with spina bifida or SCI have reduced cardiorespiratory fitness compared to non-obese typically developing children (Widman et al. 2007). Moreover, the higher the level of the impairment to the spinal cord, the greater the reduction in cardiorespiratory fitness will likely be, possibly because of the reduction in muscle mass and in heart and lung responses to exercise (Theisen 2012; West et al. 2013; Tweedy et al. 2017). The patterns seen in childhood continue in adulthood.

An evaluation of cardiorespiratory fitness can therefore provide people with spina bifida or childhood-acquired SCI, their families, and others who wish to support their health, information about whether it is low and therefore whether it may be relevant to improve cardiorespiratory fitness to help reduce risks for future poor heart health. It might also be useful to evaluate cardiorespiratory fitness if a person with spina bifida or childhood-acquired SCI or someone close to them has noted that the person physically tires more easily than in the past after physical activities including walking or manually propelling a wheelchair. Test results, in this case, can help to determine if a reduction in cardiorespiratory fitness might explain, at least in part, the change. An evaluation of cardiorespiratory fitness can also be repeated to evaluate changes over time or following an intervention.

If an evaluation of cardiorespiratory fitness (which generally uses a test to exhaustion) is not feasible for safety or practical reasons, submaximal exercise capacity might be evaluated instead. When the submaximal exercise capacity test uses a functional activity, such as walking or propelling a manual wheelchair, the test can also provide information on the capacity to do the functional activity itself, meaning a better score would indicate a better capacity to perform the task. Again, such information could be helpful if one is interested in changes over time or following an intervention or if there is concern that the capacity of the person to perform the functional activity has decreased over time.

Cardiorespiratory fitness and submaximal exercise capacity test results can also be used to help for goal-setting or motivation.

How to Evaluate the Cardiorespiratory Fitness and Submaximal Exercise Capacity of People With Spina Bifida or Childhood-Acquired SCI

How to perform these tests in general is described in Chapter 2. Additional information relevant to people with spina bifida or childhood-acquired SCI is found in this section and in Table 8.1 where examples of specific tests for this group are detailed.

Certain general safety issues to consider when performing the tests are described in Chapter 3. Safety issues specific to people with spina bifida or childhood-acquired SCI are covered in the common impairments and comorbidities sections of the present chapter. In general, because of the complex nature of spina bifida and childhood-acquired SCI, it is prudent to have medical clearance before an evaluation of cardiorespiratory fitness. In addition, the individual being tested must be able to follow simple directions to ensure the test in question can be safely and correctly performed.

LABORATORY TESTS

To accommodate for the movement difficulties of people with spina bifida or childhood-acquired SCI, laboratory tests (Table 8.1) usually start with a lower level of absolute

Table 8.1 Cardiorespiratory fitness and submaximal exercise capacity tests for people with spina bifida and childhood acquired spinal cord injury

Test	Mode	Target group	Supplementary information	References
Laboratory tests of cardiorespiratory fitness				
Adapted graded treadmill test	Treadmill walking	Children ≥6y able to walk in the community	Starting speed and speed increases depend upon walking ability as determined by the distance walked during a 6min walk test.	de Groot et al. (2011a)*
Shuttle Ride Test	Propelling a manual wheelchair	Children ≥5y who self-propel wheelchair either during daily life, long distances, or during sports (regardless of their ability to walk or not)	Considered a laboratory test when oxygen uptake is directly measured.	Bloemen et al. (2017b)*
Adaption of the McMaster All-Out Progressive Continuous Cycling Test	Cycling	People ≥14y whose main mode of mobility is walking	Must pedal at 60 revolutions/min. Starting load against which the individual pedals and increases in load every 2min are based on height. These values may have to be adjusted to ensure the tests last 8–12min. Therefore, a pre-test on a different day may be advisable.	van den Berg-Emons et al. (2003)* Bar-Or and Rowland (2004)**
Adaption of the McMaster All-Out Progressive Continuous Arm Test	Arm-cranking	People ≥14y whose main mode of mobility is self-propelling a manual wheelchair	Sits in own (immobilized) wheelchair. Must arm-crank at 60 revolutions/min. Starting load against which the individual pedals and increases in load every 2min are based on height. These values may have to be adjusted to ensure the tests last 8–12min. Therefore, a pre-test on a different day may be advisable.	van den Berg-Emons et al. (2003)* Bar-Or and Rowland (2004)**

(Continued)

Table 8.1 Continued

Test	Mode	Target group	Supplementary information	References
Field tests of cardiorespiratory fitness				
Shuttle Ride Test	Propelling a manual wheelchair	Children ≥5y who self-propel a wheelchair either during daily life, long distances, or during sports (regardless of their ability to walk or not)	Considered a field test when oxygen uptake is NOT directly measured.	Bloemen et al. (2017b)*
Test of submaximal exercise capacity				
Six-minute Walk Test	Walking	Individuals ≥6y able to walk in the community	Test can be used for those who walk but not in the community. However, if they propel a manual wheelchair for community mobility, is it probably more relevant to use the 6min push test.	de Groot et al. (2011a)*
Six-Minute Push Test	Propelling a manual wheelchair	Individuals ≥5y who self-propel a wheelchair either during daily life, long distances, or during sports (regardless of their ability to walk or not)	A practice session is recommended.	Damen et al. (2020)*

Mode: type of activity performed. Target group: target age and level of ability. References are for articles containing test instructions (*) or other key information needed to perform a test (**). Article URLs are found in the chapter reference list. Laboratory tests are typically usec in research settings or specialized clinical settings that require a measurement with a great deal of precision, otherwise field tests can be used. These latter tests can be carried out by researchers, clinicians, and other physical activity professionals. Tests are also designed for a specific target group to ensure the person performing the test has the physical abilities to perform the test correctly. With the exception of the 6min walk and ride tests, the tests were originally designed for individuals with spina bifida. They are, however, suitable for those with childhood-acquired spinal cord injury of the same target group.

physical effort, and the level of effort increases more slowly as the test goes along compared to tests for people without a health condition (van den Berg-Emons et al. 2003; Bar-Or and Rowland 2004; de Groot et al. 2011a; Bloemen et al. 2017b).

FIELD TESTS

A field test of the cardiorespiratory fitness of children with spina bifida who self-propel a manual wheelchair during daily life, long distances, or during sports (regardless of their ability to walk or not) has been developed (Table 8.1) (Bloemen et al. 2017b). It is based on the shuttle tests described in Chapter 2. A 6-minute test performed walking (de Groot et al. 2011a) or using a wheelchair (Damen et al. 2020) are the most commonly used submaximal tests (Table 8.1).

Spina Bifida- and SCI-Specific Training Principles for Cardiorespiratory Fitness

The reader is referred to Chapter 2 for an explanation of the general principles of training. Table 8.2, adapted from Tweedy et al. (2017), provides exercise guidelines for people with chronic (>6 months) spinal impairments. See De Groot et al. (2011b) for a specific training programme for children with spina bifida who walk.

It should also be noted that heart rate may be less amenable to change with training in people with spina bifida or childhood-onset SCI, especially those with higher-level lesions (i.e. where the arms as well as the legs might be affected). Medical clearance is prudent before beginning training as has been previously noted in this chapter.

MUSCULAR FITNESS (MUSCLE STRENGTH AND MUSCLE ENDURANCE)

Why Evaluate the Muscular Fitness of People With Spina Bifida or Childhood-Acquired SCI?

Chapter 2 reviews why muscular fitness is relevant to health in general. For example, poorer muscular fitness in children is associated with an increased risk profile for cardiovascular diseases in the future (García-Hermoso et al. 2019). Indeed, individuals with spina bifida demonstrate muscle weakness (Oliveira et al. 2014) as well as increased risk for cardiovascular disease (Stepanczuk et al. 2014). Therefore, similar to cardiorespiratory fitness, an evaluation of muscular fitness in the non-paralyzed muscles may provide people with spina bifida or childhood-acquired SCI, their families, clinicians, or researchers, an indication of whether or not it is low and therefore whether it may be relevant to improve muscular fitness to help reduce risks for poor cardiovascular

Table 8.2 Exercise guidelines for people with spinal cord impairment

Target	Volume of exercise	Type	Comments
Cardio-respiratory fitness	≥30min of moderate exercise on ≥5d/wk OR ≥20min of vigorous exercise on ≥3d/wk OR a combination of moderate and vigorous exercise on ≥3–5d/wk Can be accumulated in bouts of ≥10min	Exercise modes involving rhythmic contraction and relaxation of the largest available muscle groups. Examples include walking, cycling, self-propelling a manual wheelchair, arm-cranking, or swimming depending on the ability and preferences of the individual. Wheelchair users who can use their legs for exercise should be encouraged to do so to maximize the cardio-respiratory demand (intensity) and reduce the physical demand on the arms.	Moderate intensity is: - 3–6 METs - 12–13 on BRPE scale - 40–59% HRR - Able to talk but not sing Vigorous intensity is: - 6–8.8 METs - 14–15 on BRPE scale - 60–89% HRR - Only able to say a few words before needing to pause to take a breath
Muscle strength	3 sets of each exercise (1 set = 8–12 repetitions) with 2–3min recovery between each set on ≥2d/wk Moderate intensity (60–70% 1RM or 12–13 on BRPE)	Exercises should involve the major muscle groups (big muscles) and incorporate, if possible, 4–5 arm exercises. Strengthen shoulder blade stabilizers and muscles of the shoulder girdle at the back to protect against overuse injuries. Free weights, pin-loaded weights, body weight elastic bands or tubing, hydraulic resistance can be used.	The ability to contract shoulder blade stabilizers and muscles of the shoulder girdle at the back remains in people with paraplegia and progressively decreases with higher lesion level in quadriplegia. Exercises should not cause new pain. When pain is pre-existing, it should be monitored, and the exercise discontinued or modified if pain is exacerbated. Strengthen all muscles that move a joint in the different directions. To limit impingement of certain shoulder structures, avoid exercises that rotate the shoulder inwards (internal shoulder rotation) when the arm is raised to the side ≥90° (≥90° abduction).

(Continued)

Table 8.2 Continued

Target	Volume of exercise	Type	Comments
Flexibility	Hold each static stretch for 10–30s and complete 60s of total stretching time for each flexibility exercise (e.g. 2 × 30s or 4 × 15s), ≥2d/wk	Static stretching (active or passive) should be done to a point in the range where there is a feeling of tightness, slight discomfort, or, when sensation is impaired, to a point in the range at which resistance to the stretch begins to increase. Dynamic stretching can be added if possible. Stretch all major muscle groups if possible, including those of the neck, trunk, arms, and legs. Focus areas: muscles that rotate the shoulders inwards and outwards, the chest muscles, the muscles in front of the shoulder.	To limit impingement of certain shoulder structures, avoid a position that rotates the shoulder inwards (internal shoulder rotation) when completing an overhead range of motion. Stretching of paralysed muscles of the lower limbs in long-term wheelchair users should be conducted particularly cautiously due to increased incidence of a fracture risk due to low bone density (osteopenia/osteoporosis). The fingers and thumb flexors of people with quadriplegia who rely on a tenodesis grip should not be stretched.

Guidelines adapted with permission from Tweedy et al. (2016). Target: health-related fitness component targeted by the exercise. Type: examples of the types of activities; 1RM: 1 repetition maximum (see Chapter 2 for a definition); BRPE: Borg rating of perceived exertion (for rating scale see https://www.physio-pedia.com/Borg_Rating_Of_Perceived_Exertion); HRR: heart rate reserve (difference between the person's resting heart rate and their maximum heart rate, with maximum heart rate determined during a laboratory of field test of cardiorespiratory fitness); Paraplegia: weakness in the legs, due to a lesion (damage) in the thoracic (mid-back) spinal level or lower; Quadriplegia: a consequence of injuries resulting in deficits in all four limbs. Static stretch: the joint remains in one position for the stretch; Dynamic stretch: the individual contracts their muscles to move the joint through its full range to stretch the tissues; Tenodesis grip: cocking the wrist up to bend the fingers and thumb into the palm; MET: metabolic equivalent; 1 MET is the amount of energy expended when sitting quietly.

health in the future. Muscular fitness can also be reassessed to determine the effects of an intervention.

Regular evaluation of muscular fitness can also be used to determine if changes over time are affecting function. For example, one could determine if a decrease in leg muscle strength might explain a decrease in walking abilities (Schoenmakers et al. 2005). Another, perhaps even more important, reason to have regular evaluations of muscle strength over time is that muscle strength losses can be a sign of new or worsening neurological problems detailed previously in this chapter such as tethered cord, hydrocephalus, or brainstem compromise from herniation of the Chiari II malformation in spina bifida.

How to Evaluate the Muscular Fitness (Muscle Strength and Muscle Endurance) of People With Spina Bifida or Childhood-Acquired SCI

LABORATORY TESTS

Muscle strength can be measured with a specialized device that supports the arm or leg and determines the arc of movement (Widman et al. 2007), as described in Chapter 2. Children may need specialized attachments due to the size of their arms and legs (Gaul 1995). A practice session is often recommended so the individual learns what is required of them (Baltzopoulos and Kellis 1998) and two to four trials are needed to obtain a maximal result (Gaul 1995). For people with spina bifida or childhood-acquired SCI who have marked limitations to their joint movements, deformities to their arms and legs, or very weak muscles, it may not be feasible to use this method, however. In these situations, a field test may be the more appropriate option. **Muscle endurance** of the arms in individuals without extreme arm muscle weakness or marked deformities to arm joints can be measured using the arm-cranking Wingate Anaerobic test (Bloemen et al. 2017a) as described in Chapter 2. See Bloemen et al. (2017a) for test instructions.

FIELD TESTS

Muscle strength can be measured using manual muscle testing or hand-held dynamometry protocols (Mahony et al. 2009). These tests are explained in general in Chapter 2. Hand-held dynamometry is recommended if the muscles are sufficiently strong to move the arm or leg against gravity; otherwise, manual muscle testing should be used (Mahony et al. 2009). Note that for hand-held dynamometry, it is also recommended that the evaluator (often a physical therapist) be experienced with the method. See Hebert et al. (2015) for directions for using a hand-held dynamometer. The authors also provide results from this hand-held dynamometer test for a large group of typically developing children aged 4 to 17 years old. Values for a child or adolescent with spina bifida or childhood-acquired SCI can be compared to the reference values for their age and sex to help determine if weakness exists. One limitation of hand-held dynamometry, however, is that it cannot be used to measure **calf muscle strength**. In this case two options are proposed. For individuals with minor spinal cord impairment who can stand on one leg and raise up the heel of the foot, a functional test (unilateral heel rise test) can be used (Yocum et al. 2010). For all others, manual muscle testing can be used. A description of the unilateral heel rise test is given in Chapter 6. **Muscle endurance** of the arms in individuals ≥5 years who propel a manual wheelchair during daily life, long distances, or during sports (regardless of their ability to walk or not), can be evaluated using the Muscle Power Sprint test (Bloemen et al. 2017a). See Bloemen et al. (2017a) for the test directions.

Spina Bifida- and Childhood-Acquired SCI-Specific Muscular Fitness Training Principles

MUSCLE STRENGTH-SPECIFIC TRAINING PRINCIPLES

Exercise strengthening programmes can result in improvements in muscle strength in the arm and leg muscles (Andrade et al. 1991). For example, muscle strength significantly increased after a 10-week exercise training protocol that included 90 minutes of aerobic and strength exercises once a week for children with spina bifida (Andrade et al. 1991). In addition, enrolment and participation in sport activities has been shown to be associated with better muscle strength (Buffart et al. 2008). Resistance training can be used to improve strength in the non-paralyzed muscles of individuals with spina bifida or childhood-acquired SCI, similar to what is seen in people without a health condition. Chapter 2 details general training principles. Table 8.2 provides specific muscle strength training protocols for individuals with spinal cord impairment. Current best practice for increasing strength in partially paralyzed muscle includes adaptations to established strength training exercises. Recommendations are to commence with unresisted, gravity-eliminated movements, progressing, if possible, to gravity-opposed movements, and then to gravity-opposed with resistance (Harvey 2008). The programme should be supervised by a physical activity professional with experience with strength training with this group to ensure the training is performed correctly for optimum results and to avoid injury.

MUSCLE ENDURANCE-SPECIFIC TRAINING PRINCIPLES

In general, the principles as laid out in Chapter 2 apply to people with spina bifida or childhood-acquired SCI who have sufficient movement abilities to perform the training activities. The programme should be supervised by a physical activity professional with experience with this type of training with this group to ensure the feasibility of the training, to apply the correct parameters, and to avoid injury. However, very little is known about the effects of only muscle endurance training for this group.

BODY COMPOSITION

Why Evaluate the Body Composition of People With Spina Bifida or Childhood-Acquired SCI?

See Chapter 2 for a definition and a general discussion on the relevance of body composition to health. In people with spinal cord impairment, there is relative deficit in lean tissue (which is primarily skeletal muscle mass) (Liusuwan et al. 2007). For children with spina bifida this increases with age beyond 4 years, owing to segmental slowing of growth of the limbs involved (Shepherd et al. 1991). The decrease in skeletal muscle mass seen below the level of injury translates to a need for fewer calories (less energy) to maintain bodily functions, resulting in an increased risk of obesity. Overall, people with spina bifida have a higher percentage of body fat than individuals without health conditions (Oliveira et al. 2014). Adults with spina bifida in particular have a higher prevalence of obesity (Crytzer et al. 2013).

Increase in intramuscular fat is also seen. Significant changes also occur in body composition after SCI. These may have long-term health implications. Within a few weeks of injury, and up to 12 months post-injury, individuals with complete or incomplete SCI will show skeletal muscle atrophy (decrease in muscle size) below the level of injury (Castro et al. 1999; Shah et al. 2006; Gorgey and Dudley 2007). This means they will also have a deficit in muscle mass and they may be more prone to type 2 diabetes and obesity (O'Brien and Gorgey 2016).

Therefore, similar to cardiorespiratory and muscular fitness, an evaluation of body composition may provide people with spina bifida or childhood-acquired SCI, their families, clinicians, or researchers, an indication of whether or not the person is overweight or obese and therefore whether it is relevant to intervene to improve body composition to reduce risks for diseases such as cardiovascular disease or type 2 diabetes. In addition, an evaluation can be performed again after the intervention to determine its effect.

How to Evaluate the Body Composition of People With Spina Bifida or Childhood-Acquired SCI

LABORATORY TESTS

The criterion standard for measuring body composition is a full-body dual-energy X-ray absorptiometry scan (for details see Chapter 2). Percent trunk fat on dual-energy X-ray absorptiometry and abdominal girth are the most accurate ways of classifying obesity and body composition in individuals with spinal pathology (Kim et al. 2015; Liu et al. 2018).

FIELD TESTS

Waist circumference is a simple measurement performed with a flexible tape placed horizontally at the level of the umbilicus (belly button). Increasing central adiposity (fat), as measured by waist circumference, is associated with an increased risk of disease and death across multiple populations and may be suitable for identification of risk of diseases related to metabolic syndrome (described previously in this chapter) in persons with spinal cord impairment. Measurement can be done in the morning, as changes after meals may affect abdominal girth. This can be done easily at home or in a clinic setting to monitor changes and provide information on abdominal adiposity. Spina bifida and childhood-acquired SCI-specific cut points for determining overweight and obese status do not yet exist, so one can use values from the general population for an estimate. For children, one can use the following charts to determine what centile the waist circumference is closest for the child's age and sex (waist percentiles for boys 5–19 years old see https://cpeg-gcep.net/sites/default/files/upload/bookfiles/WC_M_Dec2015.pdf; waist percentile for girls 5-19 years old see https://cpeg-gcep.net/sites/default/files/upload/bookfiles/WC_F_Dec2015.pdf). As with other reference values organized as centiles (percentiles), a centile of 50 for a specific child would mean 50% of children have a waist circumference below the child's value. A child could be considered obese if their waist circumference is at or above the 93rd centile for their age and sex (Sharma et al. 2015). They could be considered overweight if it is at or above the 75th centile (but not at or above the 93rd) (Sharma et al. 2015).

For adults, the criterion is the waist circumference itself (Ross et al. 2020). Obesity is defined as a waist circumference of ≥105cm for females and ≥110cm for males. Overweight for females is defined as ≥90cm (except if ≥105 cm) and for males it is ≥100cm (except if ≥110cm).

The body mass index (described in Chapter 2) is a simple method but not accurate for people with spina bifida or childhood-acquired SCI because of the difficulty of measuring height accurately (McDonald et al. 2007). In fact, body mass index values used to calculate the risk of diseases related to obesity will underestimate the risk profile in children and adults with spinal cord pathology (Liu et al. 2018).

Effects of Physical Activity on the Body Composition of People With Spina Bifida or Childhood-Acquired SCI

Sixteen weeks of a physical activity programme (cardiorespiratory fitness training as noted in Table 8.1) may be accompanied by positive changes in body composition and increases the need for more calories (more energy) to maintain bodily functions in adults with SCI (Gorgey et al. 2016). However, these positive changes are not preserved 2 years 6 months after exercise cessation (Gorgey et al. 2016), meaning improvements that translate into better fitness and decreased risks of metabolic syndrome are not maintained if the exercise training is not maintained. For children with spina bifida who walk, a shorter aerobic exercise programme (12 weeks) did not result in changes to body composition (De Groot et al. 2011b). Whether age or the length of the programme or differences between the groups or the method of measuring body composition (only the adult study measured body composition using the criterion standard dual-energy X-ray absorptiometry), or even a combination of two or more of these factors explains the differences between the results for the two studies cannot be determined at this point. However, it should also not be surprising that physical activity or exercise alone may not always affect body composition. It has been shown that for people with spina bifida, body composition is not only related to physical activity or sedentary behaviour, but also to nutrition needs, diet, and the social and physical environment in which they live (Polfuss et al. 2017). Thus, any approach to improving body composition in people with spina bifida or childhood-acquired SCI needs to be long-term and consider physical activity behaviour as well as nutrition and environmental supports to foster an ongoing healthy diet and physically active lifestyle (McPherson et al. 2016).

FLEXIBILITY

Why Evaluate the Flexibility of People With Spina Bifida or Childhood-Acquired SCI?

See Chapter 2 for a definition and a general discussion on the relevance of flexibility to health.

People with spina bifida or childhood-acquired SCI often have imbalances in the strength of muscles around a given joint. This can result in either too much or too little flexibility. In addition, some individuals with spinal cord impairment may lack sensation including pain sensation and how extended or not a joint is (proprioception). Some people may also have an increased risk of bone fracture if they have a vitamin D deficiency, if they do not walk, are undernourished, or if they take medication for seizures. Thus, an evaluation of flexibility should be done by a qualified health care provider after an evaluation of mobility and overall health. Such a combined evaluation can provide the individual, their families, clinicians, or researchers an indication of what muscles lack flexibility, which muscles are 'lax', the impact of any flexibility on function as well as what are safe limits to the motion of the joints for flexibility and exercise training to avoid injuries (i.e. full or partial joint dislocation, broken bone). This information can then be used to design safe flexibility interventions when it is required as well as safe exercise interventions. Ongoing flexibility evaluation can be used to determine changes over time (e.g. if there is improvement or a decrease in sitting and standing posture, positioning, and walking patterns, as these may indirectly affect flexibility) or after an intervention targeting flexibility. The following are some concrete examples of flexibility issues for people with spina bifida or childhood-acquired SCI and the role of a flexibility evaluation:

- In an individual with tight knee extensors (muscles that straighten the knee) and lax knee flexors (muscles that bend the knee), an appropriate goal could be to improve flexibility in the tight knee extensors and thereby increase the ability of the knee to bend. In this case, however, it would not be appropriate to design an intervention to improve the ability of the knee to straighten, given the muscles involved (the knee flexors) are already lax.

- For people with hand weakness, some extra stiffness and partial lack of flexibility in the muscles that bend the fingers can help with functional handgrip, that is the person can cock their wrist upward, putting tension on the tissues that bend the fingers, helping to reinforce a functional grip (known as 'tenodesis'). The key here would be ongoing evaluation of flexibility of the muscles of the wrist and hand to ensure that any intervention helps rather than hinders function.

- In other situations, the evaluation of flexibility and its impact on mobility will help to determine if compromises in flexibility interventions are required depending on the overall needs of the person, as sometimes a lack of flexibility in one direction is a benefit for certain activities and not for others. For example, knees and hips that bend and stay bent in a sitting position can make sitting easier. However, if those joints do not also straighten easily, standing or lying positioning can be difficult. Sometimes a lack of flexibility itself can lead to partial or full dislocation of a joint or skin breakdown (e.g. in a foot that rolls in or out a great deal). These are examples of where it is important for individuals with spina bifida or childhood-acquired SCI and their family to work with their health care professional to determine an appropriate flexibility programme to best meet the person's needs.

How to Evaluate the Flexibility of People With Spina Bifida or Childhood-Acquired SCI

Laboratory Tests

Electrogoniometers (see Chapter 2) can be used for people with spinal cord impairment (Stein et al. 1996).

Field Tests

Flexibility is most often measured with a manual goniometer (Ekstrand et al. 1982; Al-Oraibi et al. 2013) as described in general in Chapter 2.

Effects of Physical Activity on the Flexibility of People With Spina Bifida or Childhood-Acquired SCI

General guidelines to improve flexibility training can be found in Chapter 2. Table 8.2 provides some additional information for individuals with spinal cord impairment. All flexibility (stretching) techniques should be designed to optimize stretch in the target tissue and minimize stress on other structures. Sometimes positioning devices such as braces can be used to stretch during sleeping. The programme should be individualized and designed by a qualified health care professional. In some cases, medical treatment (e.g. serial casting, medication, or surgery) may have to occur before or along with a flexibility programme, for example, when spasticity is present. Information on whether being more physically active affects flexibility for this group is lacking (Oliveira et al. 2014).

PROMOTING A PHYSICALLY ACTIVE LIFESTYLE FOR PEOPLE WITH SPINA BIFIDA OR CHILDHOOD-ACQUIRED SCI

This section on promoting a physically active lifestyle begins with a brief overview of the benefits of physical activity. A review of safety considerations is then provided, followed by some examples of feasible activities. The section ends with some information about sustaining a physically activity lifestyle. Chapters of this book that provide more general information applicable to individuals with spina bifida or childhood-acquired SCI are also referenced. For example, readers are referred to Chapter 4 for information on measuring physical activity.

Benefits of Physical Activity

The benefits to physical and mental health of exercise and a physically activity lifestyle in general have been covered in Chapters 1 and 2 as well as in the present chapter in the sections for the different components of health-related fitness. Furthermore, although people with spina bifida overall report lower levels of physical health than their peers without a health condition, those with spina bifida who have higher levels of physical activity and cardiorespiratory fitness report better physical health than those who report lower levels (Buffart et al. 2009). More physically active and fit individuals with spina bifida may also show higher levels of mental health, but the results are less conclusive (Buffart et al. 2009). Adults with spinal cord impairment who are physically active may also have a lower risk for diabetes (Itodo et al. 2022), and they appear to show better mental health and reduced chronic pain (Todd et al. 2021).

Safety Considerations

Safety considerations in general are covered in Chapter 3 and specifically for people with spina bifida or childhood-acquired SCI in the common impairments and comorbidities sections. Because individuals with spina bifida or childhood-acquired SCI are at risk of musculoskeletal, neurological, and other complications during growth and development, they should be closely monitored by their health care team to assess changes over time and provide guidance to minimize risk for these complications. In addition, physical activity professionals, families, and the individual should be aware of the specific issues for a given individual that could compromise safety and the individual should see their health care professional for evaluation quickly if symptoms appear during physical training or activity. Other methods to address specific challenges for this group to ensure safety have also been covered in this chapter under the training principles for the different components of health-related fitness.

In addition, higher levels of obesity and lower levels of fitness may predispose individuals with spinal cord impairment who engage in sports to sports-related injury such as repetitive strain, tendonitis, fracture, or shoulder injury. Therefore, prior to initiating a specific exercise or sports programme or generally increasing physical activity, at any age the individual with spina bifida or childhood-acquired SCI (and the family depending on the person's situation) should consult with their health care team to help in selecting an appropriate routine that can be done safely including if a specific conditioning programme should be established before engaging in a particular physical activity or sports programme (Murphy and Carbone 2008) or if specific techniques are required to ensure that the activity or sport is performed safely. In addition, families and physical activity professionals working with the individual should ensure that any adaptive and safety equipment is evaluated on a regular basis, as has been previously mentioned in this chapter.

Examples of Potentially Feasible Activities

The activity must be one that the individual is able to do and enjoys doing. Here are some examples of activities and for whom they would be feasible.

WALKING

This is a frequent form of exercise and physical activity. For people with spina bifida or childhood-acquired SCI who can walk, it can be used as an activity to help maintain the different components of health-related fitness mentioned in this chapter as well as helping to improve posture, skin health (through reducing pressure on the skin as can be seen with prolonged sitting and improving circulation), mood and social interactions (from being in a standing rather than sitting posture), digestion, and bowel and bladder health. The individual can walk overground (with or without a walking aid, depending on their situation and preference), or on a treadmill if they have access to one. Treadmill walking can be made easier by using a suspended harness to take some of the body weight or made more challenging by having the person walk 'uphill' by inclining the treadmill. For safety, treadmill waking is often supervised by a physical activity professional or family member trained in this. A moderate intensity walk would be one where the individual can talk but not sing.

ARM ACTIVITIES

When walking is not possible or if there may be a strong risk of injury or if it is not a preferred activity, arm activities can be considered (Theisen 2012). Arm cycling is a commonly used mode of physical activity. Intensity can be increased by arm-cranking faster and/or adding resistance to the wheel (i.e. going uphill or if using a device in a gym, by adding resistance to the fly wheel). Circuit training with arm cycling and muscle strengthening can also be used (Andrade et al. 1991; Jacobs et al. 2001). The person may also wish to use an arm-powered cycling device designed to be used for transportation.

Sports

The physical, social, and cognitive advantages of physical activity, and particularly sports and team sports, are well documented. The authors recommend that parents expose their child to a variety of sports or physical activities by age 8 or 9 years, taking into consideration the social, cognitive, and physical abilities of the child. Parents can consult with relevant members of their child's health care team and interview sport leaders and coaches to help determine if a certain programme is a good 'fit' for their child. The benefits of camp settings to improve self-care and independence are also well documented (American Camp Association 2000). These may include outdoor physical activity, organized sports, and open recreational time to connect with peers.

Sustaining an Active Lifestyle

The general approach to a sustainable, physically active lifestyle is discussed in Chapter 5 and applies to people with spina bifida or childhood-acquired SCI.

Often, it should be noted that after age 10 to 12 years children may decide to do specific activities that their same-sex peers and friends may prefer, and after the early teen years, young people tend to participate in a smaller variety of activities (Law et al. 2006), with goals of fitness, recreation, or to improve skills. By the high school years, young people will have determined to what extent if at all they choose to participate in physical activity. In our own clinical experience, we have noted that young people with spina bifida without community participation levels of at least one organized activity a week (outside of school or therapy) were amenable to social work intervention in the pre-teen years, but it became very difficult to change participation if they were over 16 to 18 years of age (Boudos and Mukherjee 2008) – thus the importance of starting young!

CONCLUSION

While individuals with spina bifida or SCI have some specific considerations that require a personalized physical activity programme with some level of supervision by qualified personnel, lack of physical activity can increase existing health issues or result in new ones. In this chapter we provide the readers with key information to help individuals with spina bifida or SCI be physically active.

REFERENCES

Adzick NS (2012) Fetal surgery for myelomeningocele: trials and tribulations. Isabella Forshall Lecture. *J Pediatr Surg* **47**: 273–281.

Adzick NS, Thom EA, Spong CY et al. (2011) A randomized trial of prenatal versus postnatal repair of myelomeningocele. *N Engl J Med* **364**: 993–1004.

Al-Oraibi S, Tariah HA, Alanazi A (2013) Serial casting versus stretching technique to treat knee flexion contracture in children with spina bifida: a comparative study. *J Pediatr Rehabil Med* **6**: 147–153.

Allergy & Asthma Network (2017) *Latex Free Sports Equipment List* [online]. LATEX AllergyAsthmaNetwork.org. Available at: **https://allergyasthmanetwork.org/wp-content/uploads/2020/05/latex-free-sports-equipment.pdf** [Accessed 2 July 2022].

American Camp Association (2000) Inclusive Outdoor Programs Benefit Youth [online]. Available at: **https://www.acacamps.org/article/camping-magazine/inclusive-outdoor-programs-benefit-youth** [Accessed 18 November 2022]. The article is freely available on the Internet and can be located using a search engine.

Andrade CK, Kramer J, Garber M, Longmuir P (1991) Changes in self-concept, cardiovascular endurance and muscular strength of children with spina bifida aged 8 to 13 years in response to a 10-week physical-activity programme: a pilot study. *Child Care Health Dev* **17**: 183–196.

Baltzopoulos V, Kellis E (1998) Isokinetic strength during childhood and adolescence. In: Van Praagh E, editor, *Pediatric Anaerobic Performance*. Champaign, IL: Human Kinetics, pp 225–240.

Bar-Or O, Rowland TW (2004) *Pediatric Exercise Medicine: From Physiologic Principles to Health Care Application*. Champaign, IL: Human Kinetics. Tables II.3 (page 348) and II.6 (page 349) provide the details for the McMaster All-Out Progressive Continuous Cycling and Arm-Cranking Tests, respectively. As URLs can change, search in Google Books for the title. Once on the book's web page in Google Books, search for the relevant table in the preview.

Bauer SB (2003) The management of the myelodysplastic child: a paradigm shift. *BJU Int* **92**: 23–28.

Bhambhani Y (2002) Physiology of wheelchair racing in athletes with spinal cord injury. *Sports Med* **32**: 23–51.

Bilston LE, Brown J (2007) Pediatric spinal injury type and severity are age and mechanism dependent. *Spine (Phila Pa 1976)* **32**: 2339–2347.

Bloemen MA, Takken T, Backx FJ, Vos M, Kruitwagen CL, De Groot JF (2017a) Validity and reliability of skill-related fitness tests for wheelchair-using youth with spina bifida. *Arch Phys Med Rehabil* **98**: 1097–1103. **https://www.archives-pmr.org/action/showPdf?pii=S0003-9993%2816%2930961-3**.

Bloemen MAT, De Groot JF, Backx FJG, Benner J, Kruitwagen C, Takken T (2017b) Wheelchair shuttle test for assessing aerobic fitness in youth with spina bifida: validity and reliability. *Phys Ther* **97**: 1020–1029. **https://www.ncbi.nlm.nih.gov/pmc/articles/PMC5803772/**.

Boudos RM, Mukherjee S (2008) Barriers to community participation: teens and young adults with spina bifida. *J Pediatr Rehabil Med* **1**: 303–310.

Buffart LM, Van den Berg-Emons RJ, Van Meeteren J, Stam HJ, Roebroeck ME (2009) Lifestyle, participation, and health-related quality of life in adolescents and young adults with myelomeningocele. *Dev Med Child Neurol* **51**: 886–894.

Buffart LM, Van der Ploeg HP, Bauman AE et al. (2008) Sports participation in adolescents and young adults with myelomeningocele and its role in total physical activity behaviour and fitness. *J Rehabil Med* **40**: 702–708.

Cardona-Grau D, Chiang G (2017) Evaluation and lifetime management of the urinary tract in patients with myelomeningocele. *Urol Clin North Am* **44**: 391–401.

Castro MJ, Apple Jr DF, Hillegass EA, Dudley GA (1999) Influence of complete spinal cord injury on skeletal muscle cross-sectional area within the first 6 months of injury. *Eur J Appl Physiol Occup Physiol* **80**: 373–378.

Crytzer TM, Dicianno BE, Kapoor R (2013) Physical activity, exercise, and health-related measures of fitness in adults with spina bifida: a review of the literature. *PM R* **5**: 1051–1062.

Damen KMS, Takken T, De Groot JF et al. (2020) 6-minute push test in youth who have spina bifida and who self-propel a wheelchair: reliability and physiologic response. *Phys Ther* **100**: 1852–1861. **https://academic.oup.com/ptj/article/100/10/1852/5870273.**

De Groot JF, Takken T, Gooskens RH et al. (2011a) Reproducibility of maximal and submaximal exercise testing in 'normal ambulatory' and 'community ambulatory' children and adolescents with spina bifida: which is best for the evaluation and application of exercise training? *Phys Ther* **91**: 267–276. **https://academic.oup.com/ptj/article/91/2/267/2735024.**

De Groot JF, Takken T, Van Brussel M et al. (2011b) Randomized controlled study of home-based treadmill training for ambulatory children with spina bifida. *Neurorehabil Neural Repair* **25**: 597–606. **https://journals.sagepub.com/doi/pdf/10.1177/1545968311400094.**

Ekstrand J, Wiktorsson M, Oberg B, Gillquist J (1982) Lower extremity goniometric measurements: a study to determine their reliability. *Arch Phys Med Rehabil* **63**: 171–175.

Eldahan KC, Rabchevsky AG (2017) Autonomic dysreflexia after spinal cord injury: systemic pathophysiology and methods of management. *Auton Neurosci* **209**: 59–70.

Garcia AM, Dicianno BE (2011) The frequency of lymphedema in an adult spina bifida population. *Am J Phys Med Rehabil* **90**: 89–96.

García-Hermoso A, Ramírez-Campillo R, Izquierdo M (2019) Is muscular fitness associated with future health benefits in children and adolescents? A systematic review and meta-analysis of longitudinal studies. *Sports Medicine* **49**: 1079–1094.

Gaul CA (1995) Muscular strength and endurance. In: Docherty D, editor, *Measurement in Pediatric Exercise Science.* Champaign, IL: Human Kinetics.

Gorgey AS, Dudley GA (2007) Skeletal muscle atrophy and increased intramuscular fat after incomplete spinal cord injury. *Spinal Cord* **45**: 304–309.

Gorgey AS, Martin H, Metz A, Khalil RE, Dolbow DR, Gater DR (2016) Longitudinal changes in body composition and metabolic profile between exercise clinical trials in men with chronic spinal cord injury. *J Spinal Cord Med* **39**: 699–712.

Hampton LE, Fletcher JM, Cirino PT et al. (2011) Hydrocephalus status in spina bifida: an evaluation of variations in neuropsychological outcomes. *J Neurosurg Pediatr* **8**: 289–298.

Harvey L (2008) *Management of Spinal Cord Injuries: A Guide for Physiotherapists.* Edinburgh: Butterworth-Heinemann.

Hebert LJ, Maltais DB, Lepage C, Saulnier J, Crete M (2015) Hand-held dynamometry isometric torque reference values for children and adolescents. *Pediatr Phys Ther* **27**: 414–423.

Henriksson H, Henriksson P, Tynelius P et al. (2020) Cardiorespiratory fitness, muscular strength, and obesity in adolescence and later chronic disability due to cardiovascular disease: a cohort study of 1 million men. *European Heart Journal* **41**: 1503–1510.

Itodo OA, Flueck JL, Raguindin PF et al. (2022) Physical activity and cardiometabolic risk factors in individuals with spinal cord injury: a systematic review and meta-analysis. *Eur J Epidemiol* **37**: 335–365.

Jacobs PL, Nash MS, Rusinowski JW (2001) Circuit training provides cardiorespiratory and strength benefits in persons with paraplegia. *Med Sci Sports Exerc* **33**: 711–717.

Juranek J, Dennis M, Cirino PT, El-Messidi L, Fletcher JM (2010) The cerebellum in children with spina bifida and Chiari II malformation: quantitative volumetrics by region. *Cerebellum* **9**: 240–248.

Kim SG, Ko K, Hwang IC, Suh HS, Kay S, Caterson I, Kim KK (2015) Relationship between indices of obesity obtained by anthropometry and dual-energy X-ray absorptiometry: The Fourth and Fifth Korea National Health and Nutrition Examination Survey (KNHANES IV and V, 2008–2011). *Obes Res Clin Pract* **9**: 487–498.

Lala D, Craven BC, Thabane L et al. (2014) Exploring the determinants of fracture risk among individuals with spinal cord injury. *Osteoporos Int* **25**: 177–185.

Law M, King G, King S et al. (2006) Patterns of participation in recreational and leisure activities among children with complex physical disabilities. *Dev Med Child Neurol* **48**: 337–342.

Leibold S, Ekmark E, Adams RC (2000) Decision-making for a successful bowel continence program. *Eur J Pediatr Surg* **10**: 26–30.

Liu JS, Dong C, Vo AX et al. (2018) Obesity and anthropometry in spina bifida: what is the best measure. *J Spinal Cord Med* **41**: 55–62.

Liusuwan RA, Widman LM, Abresch RT, Styne DM, McDonald CM (2007) Body composition and resting energy expenditure in patients aged 11 to 21 years with spinal cord dysfunction compared to controls: comparisons and relationships among the groups. *J Spinal Cord Med,* 30 Suppl 1: S105–S111.

Mahony K, Hunt A, Daley D, Sims S, Adams R (2009) Inter-tester reliability and precision of manual muscle testing and hand-held dynamometry in lower limb muscles of children with spina bifida. *Phys Occup Ther Pediatr* **29**: 44–59.

Mazzeo F, Santamaria S, Iavarone A (2015) 'Boosting' in Paralympic athletes with spinal cord injury: doping without drugs. *Funct Neurol* **30**: 91–98.

McDonald CM, Abresch-Meyer AL, Nelson MD, Widman LM (2007) Body mass index and body composition measures by dual X-ray absorptiometry in patients aged 10 to 21 years with spinal cord injury. *J Spinal Cord Med* **30**: S97–104.

McPherson AC, Ball GD, Maltais DB et al. (2016) A call to action: Setting the research agenda for addressing obesity and weight-related topics in children with physical disabilities. *Child Obes* **12**: 59–69.

Murphy NA, Carbone PS (2008) Promoting the participation of children with disabilities in sports, recreation, and physical activities. *Pediatrics* **121**: 1057–1061.

O'Brien LC, Gorgey AS (2016) Skeletal muscle mitochondrial health and spinal cord injury. *World J Orthop* **7**: 628–637.

Oliveira A, Jacome C, Marques A (2014) Physical fitness and exercise training on individuals with spina bifida: a systematic review. *Res Dev Disabil* **35**: 1119–1136.

Oomman A (2013) Latex glove allergy: the story behind the 'invention' of the surgical glove and the emergence of latex allergy. *Archives of International Surgery* **3**: 201–204.

Pandey A, Gupta V, Singh SP, Kumar V, Verma R (2015) Neuropathic ulcers among children with neural tube defects: a review of literature. *Ostomy Wound Manage* **61**: 32–38.

Parker SE, Mai CT Canfield MA et al. (2010) Updated National Birth Prevalence estimates for selected birth defects in the United States, 2004–2006. *Birth Defects Res A Clin Mol Teratol* **88**: 1008–1016.

Perez M, Lemelle JL, Barthelme H, Marquand D, Schmitt M (2001) Bowel management with antegrade colonic enema using a Malone or a Monti conduit: clinical results. *Eur J Pediatr Surg* **11**: 315–318.

Polfuss M, Bandini LG, Sawin KJ (2017) Obesity prevention for individuals with spina bifida. *Curr Obes Rep* **6**: 116–126.

Ross R, Neeland IJ, Yamashita S et al. (2020) Waist circumference as a vital sign in clinical practice: a Consensus Statement from the IAS and ICCR Working Group on Visceral Obesity. *Nat Rev Endocrinol* **16**: 177–189.

Ruiz JR, Castro-Pinero J, Artero EG et al. (2009) Predictive validity of health-related fitness in youth: a systematic review. *Br J Sports Med* **43**: 909–923.

Schluer AB, Cignacco E, Muller M, Halfens RJ (2009) The prevalence of pressure ulcers in four paediatric institutions. *J Clin Nurs* **18**: 3244–3252.

Schoenmakers MA, Uiterwaal CS, Gulmans VA, Gooskens RH, Helders PJ (2005) Determinants of functional independence and quality of life in children with spina bifida. *Clin Rehabil* **19**: 677–685.

Selvarajah S, Schneider EB, Becker D, Sadowsky CL, Haider AH, Hammond ER (2014) The epidemiology of childhood and adolescent traumatic spinal cord injury in the United States: 2007–2010. *J Neurotrauma* **31**: 1548–1560.

Shah PK, Stevens JE, Gregory CM et al. (2006) Lower-extremity muscle cross-sectional area after incomplete spinal cord injury. *Arch Phys Med Rehabil* **87**: 772–778.

Sharma AK, Metzger DL, Daymont C, Hadjiyannakis S, Rodd CJ (2015) LMS tables for waist-circumference and waist-height ratio Z-scores in children aged 5–19y in NHANES III: association with cardio-metabolic risks. *Pediatr Res* **78**: 723–729.

Shepherd K, Roberts D, Golding S, Thomas BJ, Shepherd RW (1991) Body composition in myelomeningocele. *Am J Clin Nutr* **53**: 1–6.

Stein RB, Zehr EP, Lebiedowska MK, Popovic DB, Scheiner A, Chizeck HJ (1996) Estimating mechanical parameters of leg segments in individuals with and without physical disabilities. *IEEE Trans Rehabil Eng* **4**: 201–211.

Stepanczuk BC, Dicianno BE, Webb TS (2014) Young adults with spina bifida may have higher occurrence of prehypertension and hypertension. *Am J Phys Med Rehabil* **93**: 200–206.

Symonds A, Barbareschi G, Taylor S, Holloway C (2018) A systematic review: the influence of real time feedback on wheelchair propulsion biomechanics. *Disabil Rehabil Assist Technol* **13**: 47–53.

Theisen D (2012) Cardiovascular determinants of exercise capacity in the Paralympic athlete with spinal cord injury. *Exp Physiol* **97**: 319–324.

Todd KR, Lawrason SVC, Shaw RB, Wirtz D, Martin Ginis KA (2021) Physical activity interventions, chronic pain, and subjective well-being among persons with spinal cord injury: a systematic scoping review. *Spinal Cord* **59**: 93–104.

Tweedy SM, Beckman EM, Geraghty TJ et al. (2017) Exercise and sports science Australia (ESSA) position statement on exercise and spinal cord injury. *J Sci Med Sport* **20**: 108–115.

Van den Berg-Emons HJ, Bussmann JB, Meyerink HJ, Roebroeck ME, Stam HJ (2003) Body fat, fitness and level of everyday physical activity in adolescents and young adults with meningomyelocele. *J Rehabil Med* **35**: 271–275. **https://www.medicaljournals.se/jrm/content/abstract/10.1080/16501970310012400**.

Vanhala M, Vanhala P, Kumpusalo E, Halonen P, Takala J (1998) Relation between obesity from childhood to adulthood and the metabolic syndrome: population based study. *BMJ* **317**: 319.

West CR, Bellantoni A, Krassioukov AV (2013) Cardiovascular function in individuals with incomplete spinal cord injury: a systematic review. *Top Spinal Cord Inj Rehabil* **19**: 267–278.

Widman LM, Abresch RT, Styne DM, McDonald CM (2007) Aerobic fitness and upper extremity strength in patients aged 11 to 21 years with spinal cord dysfunction as compared to ideal weight and overweight controls. *J Spinal Cord Med* **30**: S88–96.

Yocum A, McCoy SW, Bjornson KF, Mullens P, Burton GN (2010) Reliability and validity of the standing heel-rise test. *Phys Occup Ther Pediatr* **30**: 190–204.

CHAPTER 9

Childhood-Onset Neuromuscular Conditions

Craig Campbell and Katy de Valle

This chapter begins with an overview of childhood-onset neuromuscular conditions, including common impairments, comorbidities, and medications. Next, the health-related fitness components of cardiorespiratory fitness and submaximal exercise capacity, muscular fitness, body composition, and flexibility are reviewed (see Chapter 2 for definitions of these terms). For each component, the reader is provided with information on why one might wish to evaluate it, how to evaluate it, and either training principles specific to childhood-onset neuromuscular conditions (cardiorespiratory fitness and submaximal exercise capacity, muscular fitness) or a discussion about how physical activity affects the component (body composition, flexibility). The chapter ends with an overview of guidelines to promote a physically active lifestyle for people with childhood-onset neuromuscular conditions.

A further note on health-related fitness tests – they are classed as laboratory or field tests, with laboratory tests being used more often in research or in specialized clinical contexts and field tests being used more broadly, in research, clinical, and community contexts. The reader is referred to Chapter 2 for a more detailed description of laboratory and field tests.

Throughout the chapter, when the reader is referred to resources by the statement 'see Author et al. (year)' or when article URLs are mentioned in the table legends, that means the article or document cited is freely available on the internet and the URL or other information needed to locate the article or document is found following the corresponding reference in the reference list.

WHAT ARE CHILDHOOD-ONSET NEUROMUSCULAR CONDITIONS?

Childhood-onset neuromuscular conditions affect muscles and related functions because of problems with the peripheral nervous system (the nervous system outside the brain and the spinal cord) and the muscles themselves. Individuals with childhood-onset neuromuscular conditions can have difficulty walking, limited flexibility and range of joint motion (contractures), a curved spine (scoliosis), and respiratory failure. With peripheral nerve conditions, there is also an element of sensory loss that compromises functioning over and above the muscle weakness. These impairments are frequently associated with significant lifelong morbidities (related health problems), which are often severe and can be life-limiting.

The majority of childhood-onset neuromuscular conditions have a genetic basis (Darras 2015), with the most common one being Duchenne muscular dystrophy, a muscle disease that globally affects about 7.1 per 100 000 males (Crisafulli et al. 2020). Other common childhood-onset neuromuscular conditions include spinal muscular atrophy (a disease of motor neurons, which are responsible for controlling muscle movement); myotonic dystrophy (a multi-system condition with a significant muscle component); and Charcot–Marie–Tooth disease (a condition of the peripheral nerve). As discussed below in the common medications section, no effective treatments are presently available to alter the primary causes of most childhood-onset neuromuscular conditions, apart from spinal muscular atrophy. The mainstay of all health care involves management of the secondary effects.

COMMON IMPAIRMENTS AND COMORBIDITIES

The main impairment is muscle weakness. Childhood-onset neuromuscular disorders are often accompanied by manifestations outside of those strictly related to muscle weakness. These are termed comorbidities. In some cases, such as breathing difficulties, the muscular weakness has a direct impact, but for issues such as intellectual or developmental disability, this can be an association due to alternate brain development related to the underlying genetic mutation. In some cases, the condition is progressive and the muscle weakness and related comorbidities can increase over time. For example, children with Duchenne muscular dystrophy progressively lose muscle function and eventually require a wheelchair for mobility (usually around the beginning of adolescence) and breathing support later. Death usually occurs in the 20s due to heart or breathing problems. Table 9.1 details common comorbidities and their impact according to the specific childhood-onset neuromuscular condition.

COMMON MEDICATIONS

Very few childhood-onset neuromuscular conditions have a medication that markedly changes the course of the condition, although it is an active area of novel therapy

Table 9.1 Common comorbidities and their impact on management

Childhood-onset neuromuscular condition	Comorbidities	Impact
Spinal muscular atrophy	1. Feeding dysfunction and constipation 2. Respiratory (breathing) failure 3. Autonomic storms (episodes of sweating, increased heart rate, flushing)	1. Require regular monitoring for stomach and intestine problems including weight gain and difficulty swallowing. 2. Require regular monitoring for breathing issues. 3. Require regular monitoring for autonomic issues.
Charcot–Marie–Tooth (peripheral neuropathy)	1. Pain 2. Hearing loss	1. Require pain management (can be drug or non-drug in nature). 2. Require audiology monitoring.
Duchenne muscular dystrophy	1. Developmental disability 2. Constipation 3. Scoliosis (spinal curving) 4. Heart disease 5. Respiratory (breathing) failure 6. Anxiety disorders and depression 7. Tic disorders	1–7. Require extensive monitoring, support, and treatment as needed.
Myotonic dystrophy	1. Developmental disability 2. Feeding dysfunction 3. Constipation or diarrhea 4. Heart arrhythmia (atypical heartbeat) 5. Hypothyroidism (underactive thyroid) 6. Dental issues 7. Anxiety disorders 8. Attention issues 9. Hydrocephalus in the congenital form (accumulation of fluid in the cavities in the brain)	1. Require learning assessments and coordinated academic support. 2–9. Require regular monitoring of all body systems impacted for a given comorbidity.

For each condition, the impacts are linked to their comorbidities by number.

development and an exciting and hopeful time for the neuromuscular community. New approved therapies for spinal muscular atrophy such as gene therapy and genetic-based therapy have made a dramatic change in outcome, particularly when given in the first months of life and/or before symptoms begin. In fact, the effectiveness of these treatments in altering the trajectory of spinal muscular atrophy has resulted in many countries across the globe moving toward newborn screening for the condition. In other neuromuscular diseases, drug management is focused on protecting muscle function; for example, corticosteroid use in Duchenne muscular dystrophy can reduce muscle inflammation. Various medications can also be used specifically to protect heart function. Other medication can be used to maintain health (e.g. to maintain bone health) or address symptoms that can arise, such as pain. New experimental medications are also being developed that appear to address some of the genetic mutations that lead to childhood-onset neuromuscular disorders and improve function.

CARDIORESPIRATORY FITNESS AND SUBMAXIMAL EXERCISE CAPACITY

Why Evaluate These Constructs for People With Childhood-Onset Neuromuscular Conditions?

Chapter 2 provides the definitions of cardiorespiratory fitness and submaximal exercise capacity, details the differences in general between children and adults, and describes the relevance of cardiorespiratory fitness and submaximal exercise capacity to overall health and functioning.

Overall, cardiorespiratory fitness and submaximal exercise capacity is reduced in people with childhood-onset neuromuscular conditions. Thus, cardiorespiratory fitness or submaximal exercise capacity evaluations can be performed to provide people with childhood-onset neuromuscular conditions, their families, clinicians, or researchers with information to help determine an individual's level of endurance for performing activities such as walking, or using the arms, which, in turn, can help determine what equipment they may require to support their participation and independence. An evaluation of cardiorespiratory fitness and submaximal exercise capacity can also help in determining what is a safe level of intensity for physical activities such as walking or swimming. For submaximal exercise capacity tests that use a functional activity such as walking, the test might also be used to evaluate the functional activity itself. Cardiorespiratory fitness or submaximal exercise capacity evaluations can be repeated to determine changes over time or as the result of an intervention, including medication.

How to Evaluate These Constructs for People With Childhood-Onset Neuromuscular Conditions

The following section provides information about evaluating the cardiorespiratory fitness and submaximal exercise capacity of people with childhood-onset neuromuscular conditions. Given the heart, lung, and muscle problems of these individuals, an evaluation of cardiorespiratory fitness, which requires a test to exhaustion, is generally only feasible and safe in individuals with only mild movement capacity limitations and without marked lung or heart problems as determined by their physician, meaning they have received medical clearance to be able to perform the test (Bartels et al. 2015). This will typically be younger children. When it is not feasible or safe to evaluate cardiorespiratory fitness, an evaluation of submaximal exercise capacity can be performed, again, provided that the individual has sufficient muscle, heart, and lung function to perform the test, and they have received medical clearance to be able to perform the test. Additional general safety issues for these types of tests are described in Chapter 3.

LABORATORY TESTS

Given the safety issues, these tests must be carried out by exercise professionals with experience with this type of testing with this population and following safety clearance by the individual's physician. A cycling test may be more feasible and safer than a treadmill test because there is less risk of falling. The loads against which the individual pedals should also be somewhat individualized according to their movement abilities. See Bartels et al. (2015) for specific directions for such a test to measure cardiorespiratory fitness. The assisted 6-minute cycling (or arm-cranking) test (Jansen et al. 2012; Dirks et al. 2016) can be used to measure the submaximal exercise capacity of people with childhood-onset neuromuscular conditions for whom a submaximal exercise test done by walking is longer possible but for whom submaximal exercise testing remains safe (i.e. they do not show symptoms of heart disease and they have received medical clearance) and perhaps for whom a cycling test of cardiorespiratory fitness (i.e. a test to exhaustion) is not feasible or safe. See Dirks et al. (2016) for instructions for the test. This test is considered a laboratory test because it requires specialized equipment, a stationary exercise testing device that allows for assisted (motorized) cycling or arm-cranking, and records the number of revolutions performed as well as evaluators with expertise with the test. With this test, a pre-set level of motorized assistance is used, one that the individual can maintain for 6 minutes. The test is scored as the number of revolutions performed over the 6 minutes. Rests are allowed and recorded.

FIELD TESTS

The 6-minute walk test as described in Chapter 2 is a commonly used test of submaximal exercise capacity for ambulatory individuals with childhood-onset neuromuscular conditions (McDonald et al. 2010; Montes et al. 2010). For these individuals, a 25m track can be used. Walking endurance can be estimated by measuring the reduction in speed over the test duration, that is by noting the distance walked in each of the 6 minutes (typically marked on the track). At the end of the test the distance walked in each minute is calculated and added to give a total distance walked. See Bushby and Connor (2011) for reference values for the test for children with Duchenne muscular dystrophy, which allow one to compare with results of a given child to the results for a group of children with Duchenne muscular dystrophy of the same age. In addition, for children with Duchenne muscular dystrophy, it has been shown that a result on the

6-minute walk test of <325m can indicate an increased risk for decreased walking ability over the subsequent year (McDonald et al. 2013). Thus, the results of the 6-minute walk test may also help clinicians, individuals, and families make the adaptations needed to ensure optimal participation and independence over time when walking ability is decreasing.

Childhood-Onset Neuromuscular Condition-Specific Training Principles for Cardiorespiratory Fitness

Training principles should consider frequency, intensity, time, and type as described in Chapter 2. Published literature recommends the introduction of moderate intensity exercises (those requiring a moderate amount of effort three to five times per week) early in the course of childhood-onset neuromuscular conditions, to slow functional decline, even in deteriorating conditions such as Duchenne muscular dystrophy (Jansen et al. 2013). A moderate intensity would be one where, according to the 'Talk Test', the individual can still talk out loud but not sing while training. See Utter et al. (2002) for the Children's OMNI Scale of Perceived Exertion which can also be used to determine intensity. In this case a moderate intensity would be from three to less than six. The theory of early exercise reducing the effect of disuse weakness would support this recommendation. In terms of type, a 2013 study in Duchenne muscular dystrophy reports that exercising upper and lower limbs with an assisted cycling device at a moderate intensity helps to reduce functional decline caused by disuse without side effects (Jansen et al. 2013). Jansen et al. also suggest that to maintain the positive effects of exercise, individuals must 'use it or lose it'. This is a well-known training principle across populations and may be even more important in those with childhood-onset neuromuscular conditions than in the general population. Exercise options available to muscles that are extremely weak (less than 10% of normal strength), however, are limited and their benefits are difficult to quantify (Forrest and Qian 1999). Encouraging the introduction of exercise prior to this level of deterioration gives the best chance of achieving improved function. It is important that the programme be supervised, at least at the beginning, by a professional with experience of cardiorespiratory fitness with the population in question (Voet 2019).

MUSCULAR FITNESS (MUSCLE STRENGTH AND MUSCLE ENDURANCE)

Why Evaluate the Muscular Fitness of People With Childhood-Onset Neuromuscular Conditions?

Muscle weakness (see Chapter 2 for a definition) is the hallmark of all childhood-onset neuromuscular conditions, and the cause of weakness differs depending on the particular childhood-onset neuromuscular condition. Due to the potential negative impact of muscle fatigue in childhood-onset neuromuscular conditions, it is important to measure both strength and endurance to evaluate an individual's muscular fitness effectively. Overall, an evaluation of muscular fitness can help to characterize a main component of the condition. As with cardiorespiratory fitness or submaximal exercise capacity, an evaluation of muscular fitness can be repeated to determine changes over time or as the result of an intervention, including medication.

How to Evaluate the Muscular Fitness of People With Childhood-Onset Neuromuscular Conditions

The following section provides information about evaluating the muscular fitness of people with childhood-onset neuromuscular conditions. Measurement of muscular strength in particular is complex in individuals with childhood-onset neuromuscular conditions and should be evaluated, if possible, with tests that directly measure the strength of particular muscle or muscle group as well as with tests that measure muscle strength indirectly using functional activities as described in the next section. For some individuals, depending on their level of muscle weakness, only tests more functional in nature may be feasible or safe. In addition, an indirect measure using a functional test is also often the safest and more feasible approach to measuring muscle endurance. Laboratory tests are carried out by researchers and exercise professionals with expertise with the particular test with the population in question. Field tests can be carried out by clinicians and other exercise professionals with expertise with the particular test with the population in question.

Laboratory Tests

To measure **muscle strength**: systems such as load cells or isokinetic dynamometers have been used extensively with this population, particularly during clinical trials to assess the effects of various interventions. Assessment of strength using this method has been shown to be more accurate and sensitive to change when compared to manual muscle testing. It is recognized, however, that these measures do not provide meaningful information about how a child functions in their daily life. In general, these tests cannot measure differences in a consistent manner in many children under the age of 6 years (Merlini et al. 1995). **Muscle endurance** can be evaluated using the Wingate test (Bar-Or 1996; Van Mil et al. 1996), as described in Chapter 2. It should be noted, however, that this test is rarely used in neuromuscular conditions because of concerns regarding exacerbating muscle damage given the high intensity nature of the test.

Field Tests

Muscle strength can be evaluated with manual muscle testing (see Chapter 2 for details) in childhood-onset neuromuscular conditions (Florence et al. 1985, 1992). It is quick and easy to administer, requires no additional equipment, and has demonstrated good consistency in clinicians experienced in its use, although it has a lack of sensitivity to change. It is considered a pragmatic clinical measure of muscle strength. Hand-held dynamometry as described in Chapter 2 is another method of measuring muscle strength in this population (Merlini et al. 2002). Compared to the previously mentioned laboratory test, a hand-held dynamometer has the advantage of being a relatively inexpensive, portable device that allows accurate strength measures of individual muscles or muscle groups to be taken easily in a busy clinical setting. See Hebert et al. (2015) for the test directions. As has been noted previously in this chapter, tests that measure muscle strength indirectly using functional activities should be used to complement a more direct measure of muscle strength. Frequently used functional tests for individuals with childhood-onset neuromuscular conditions are the North Star Ambulatory Assessment (Scott et al. 2012; Mayhew et al. 2013; Mercuri et al. 2016; Ricotti et al. 2016; UK North Star Clinical Network 2017), the Performance of the Upper Limb module for Duchenne muscular dystrophy (Mayhew et al. 2020), the Hammersmith Functional Motor Scale Expanded (Smartnet and PNCR 2009; Glanzman et al. 2011), the Revised Hammersmith Scale for spinal muscular atrophy (Ramsey et al. 2017), the Revised Upper Limb Module (Mazzone 2014; Mazzone et al. 2017), and the Charcot–Marie–Tooth disease Pediatric Scale (Burns and The Inherited Neuropathies Consortium 2011; Burns et al. 2012; Burns and The Inherited Neuropathies Consortium 2022). Of note, scores on the North Star Ambulatory Assessment can also be used to predict when the loss of walking abilities may start (Ricotti et al. 2016). Table 9.2 provides information on the target group for each of these tests as well as test descriptions. **Muscle endurance** tests as described in Chapter 2 are often too intense to be used safely with this group. Instead, the 6-minute walk test as described previously in this chapter and in Chapter 2 can be used to indirectly evaluate walking-related muscular endurance by evaluating the change in walking speed over the 6 minutes.

Childhood-Onset Neuromuscular Condition-Specific Principles for Strength Training

Only strength training will be addressed in the following section as the safety of endurance training as defined in Chapter 2 has not been established for this group.

At present, it is known that moderate intensity resistance training following the training guidelines in Chapter 2 in muscles without severe disease is likely to be effective in slowly progressive childhood-onset neuromuscular conditions (Forrest and Qian 1999; Kilmer 2002; White et al. 2004; Cup et al. 2007; Voet et al. 2010; Markert et al. 2012; White et al. 2014; Burns et al. 2017; Lott et al. 2021; Hammer et al. 2022).

STRENGTH TRAINING PARAMETERS

The following are some guidelines for strength training parameters (intensity, frequency, repetitions, sets, duration, target muscles). However, it is important

Table 9.2 Functional tests to indirectly evaluate muscle strength for individuals with childhood onset neuromuscular conditions

Test	Target group	Supplementary information	References
North Star Ambulatory Assessment	Males with Duchenne muscular dystrophy ≥3y who walk (test modified by omitting some items for males <4y)	Evaluates the ability to perform various activities such as standing from a sitting position, walking up and down a step, standing on one leg, jumping, and hopping. For males >7y, a score of ≤34 on the transformed scale found in Mayhew et al. (2013) indicates a risk of losing some walk ability over the following year (Ricotti et al. 2016).	UK North Star Clinical Network (2017)* Bushby and Connor (2011)** Mayhew et al. (2013)***
Performance of the Upper Limb module for Duchenne muscular dystrophy	Males with Duchenne muscular dystrophy ≥7y who walk and who do not walk	Evaluates the ability to perform various activities with the arms and hands such as lifting the arm to eye level, lifting and moving a weight from one point to another on a table, removing a lid from a standard container, tearing a piece of paper.	Mayhew et al. (2020)*
Hammersmith Functional Motor Scale Expanded and Revised Hammersmith Scale	Children and young adults with type 2 and type 3 spinal muscular atrophy ≥2y who walk and who do not walk	Evaluates the ability to perform a wide range of movement skills such as rolling, lifting the head, sitting independently, maintaining a hands and knees posture, climbing four stairs, walking, running, jumping, and hopping.	Smartnet and PNCR (2009)* Ramsey et al. (2017)*
Revised Upper Limb Module	Children and young adults with type 2 and type 3 spinal muscular atrophy ≥30mo who walk and who do not walk.	18 items of upper limb function with a 3-point scale from 0 (unable) to 2 (able with no difficulty). An additional item (Open Ziploc container) is scored as 0 (cannot) or 1 (can). There is also an item not scored, but used to assign a functional class.	Mazzone et al. (2017)* Mazzone (2014)*
Charcot–Marie–Tooth disease Pediatric Scale	Individuals 3–20y with Charcot–Marie–Tooth disease	The test contains 11 items. Muscle strength is directly evaluated in two items (grip strength and ankle strength) and indirectly evaluated through items that measure activities such as hand and finger dexterity, balance, and walking ability. One item, a sensation measure, is not a strength measure per se but relevant to this group's movement abilities, nonetheless.	Burns and The Inherited Neuropathies Consortium (2011)* Burns and The Inherited Neuropathies Consortium (2022)*

Functional tests are field tests that can be carried by researchers, clinicians, and other physical activity professionals to indirectly evaluate muscle strength through evaluating the ability to perform various physical tasks. Tests are also designed for a specific target group to ensure the person performing the test has the physical abilities to perform the test correctly, and that the physical tasks evaluated are relevant to them. Reference values for individuals are similar to the target group and can help in interpreting the test results. Type 2 and type 3 spinal muscular atrophy: these are milder forms of the condition. Individuals living with type 2 spinal muscular atrophy are able to sit, but do not stand or walk whereas individuals living with type 3 spinal muscular atrophy are able to walk when they are younger but may lose the ability as they grow older. References are for articles containing test instructions (*) or values for comparison purposes such as reference values (**) or clinically meaningful differences (***). If two references are listed for test instructions, both may be needed. Article URLs are found in the chapter reference list.

that the training programme is supervised by an exercise professional with experience with such training with the population in question to determine how the parameters might apply to a particular individual. As in the general population, the effectiveness of strengthening programmes for people with childhood-onset neuromuscular conditions will be affected by training parameters used (Markert et al. 2012) as well as the degree of weakness (Forrest and Qian 1999) and the physical abilities of the child.

Intensity

- Post-exercise soreness, muscle swelling, short-term weakness, muscle tightness, and myoglobinuria (dark-coloured urine) are signs of exercise-induced muscle damage and that the training intensity was likely too high.
- Therefore, to be prudent:
  1. Begin with light intensity training (i.e. 20–30% of the one-repetition maximum load or weight as defined in Chapter 2) for 1 or 2 weeks before increasing the intensity to moderate (i.e. 40%–50% of the one-repetition maximum load or weight as defined in Chapter 2).
  2. Exercise the muscles of one limb for the first week or two (assuming there are no signs the intensity is too high) until it can be established that the muscles can tolerate strength training.

Frequency, Repetitions, and Sets

- Start with what is on the lower end of what is recommended in Chapter 2, at least to begin with (i.e. two times per week on non-consecutive days, six repetitions per set with two sets per muscle group).

Duration

- As noted in Chapter 2, the programme should last a minimum of 8 to 20 weeks, assuming no safety issues.

Target Muscles

- This will depend on the health condition and specific needs and desires of the individual.
- By way of example:
  1. Muscles that bend and straighten the knee have been targeted for males with Duchenne muscular dystrophy (de Lateur and Giaconi 1979; Lott et al. 2021).
  2. Muscles that pull up the foot and ankle have been targeted for children with Charcot–Marie–Tooth disease (Burns et al. 2017).

BODY COMPOSITION

Why Evaluate the Body Composition of People With Childhood-Onset Neuromuscular Conditions?

Children with childhood-onset neuromuscular conditions are at risk of being either overweight, obese, or underweight depending on their particular neuromuscular condition. The risk can also change through their lifespan as the disease progresses. For example, males with Duchenne muscular dystrophy who take steroids often show excessive weight gain when they are younger, but this may change in later years when they require assistance to maintain adequate nutrition due to chewing and swallowing becoming more difficult. People with childhood-onset neuromuscular conditions also have altered body composition compared to their typically developing peers (Moore et al. 2016). Quite commonly, they have an increased body fat mass along with reduced lean muscle mass. However, this is not always evident when body composition is assessed with standard measures such as weight or body mass index (see Chapter 2 for a definition of body mass index). Increased fatty infiltration of muscles is evident in some childhood-onset neuromuscular conditions such as Duchenne muscular dystrophy (Davidson and Truby 2009), where the muscles appear enlarged.

It is important to understand body composition changes for several reasons:

- These changes can be used as a marker of disease progression (muscle mass reduces as disease progresses and this muscle is often replaced by fat).
- They give a clearer understanding of what is occurring in the context of growth (i.e. whether a child actually gained muscle over the year, or has simply gained fat mass).
- These changes are important for assessing the impact of therapeutic interventions specifically around weight management.

How to Evaluate the Body Composition of People With Childhood-Onset Neuromuscular Conditions

As with tests of other areas of health-related fitness, laboratory tests are carried out by researchers and exercise professionals with expertise with the particular test with the population in question and field tests can be carried out by clinicians and other exercise professionals with expertise with the particular test with the population in question.

LABORATORY TESTS

Several tests requiring specialized equipment are detailed in Chapter 2. By way of example, dual-energy X-ray absorptiometry can be used with individuals with childhood-onset neuromuscular conditions. Bioelectrical impedance has also been shown to give a reasonable estimate of body composition, depending on the mathematical equations used to interpret the results (Elliott et al. 2015).

Body mass index, as noted in Chapter 2, is a gross indicator and should not be relied on as the sole measure of body composition; however, it is useful within a clinical setting when more accurate laboratory tests cannot be done. Its limitations, as detailed in Chapter 2, are relevant to childhood-onset neuromuscular conditions. Body mass index in males with Duchenne muscular dystrophy will tend to underestimate their fat mass (Davidson and Truby 2009). Skin fold tests as described in Chapter 2 are another measure of body composition but have limited use for assessment in childhood-onset neuromuscular conditions as they are unable to assess fatty infiltration within muscles.

Effects of Physical Activity on the Body Composition of People With Childhood-Onset Neuromuscular Conditions

Research regarding the effects of physical activity on body composition is limited in childhood-onset neuromuscular conditions. What is known is that children with these conditions perform less physical activity compared to their peers. They typically have increased fat and reduced muscle mass. Whether decreased energy expenditure (calories burned) from reduced physical activity or a defect in energy metabolism (how calories are burned) are contributing factors to increased body adiposity fat mass in childhood-onset neuromuscular conditions is unknown. What is recommended to address overweight and obesity for children with physical disabilities in general is a holistic approach that considers both nutrition and physical activity (McPherson et al. 2016). Therefore, people with childhood-onset neuromuscular conditions who wish to address body composition issues may wish to consult with professionals in both physical activity and nutrition with experience with this group.

FLEXIBILITY

Why Evaluate the Flexibility of People With Childhood-Onset Neuromuscular Conditions?

Chapter 2 provides details on a definition of flexibility. For people with childhood-onset neuromuscular conditions, a lack of muscle and joint flexibility (seen as muscle and joint tightness) is a common secondary complication of the condition, along with muscle weakness. Tightness can be caused by factors common to all childhood-onset neuromuscular conditions including the inability to move the joints actively through their full joint range, habitual positioning, and muscle strength imbalances across joints where the different muscles weaken at different rates. Other causes may be condition-specific such as fibrotic changes (thickening and scarring of connective tissue) within the muscles seen commonly in Duchenne muscular dystrophy (Bushby et al. 2010). Maintaining muscle and joint flexibility is essential for preserving physical functions such as walking or hand function and helps avoid the development of contractures (muscle and other tissue shortening around a joint that reduces range through which the joint can move). The accurate evaluation of muscle and joint range enables the implementation of preventive strategies such as stretching, splinting, equipment prescription, or surgery in a timely manner.

How to Evaluate the Flexibility of People With Childhood-Onset Neuromuscular Conditions

LABORATORY TESTS

X-rays are the primary laboratory-based assessment for flexibility where there are fixed deformities that are impacting bone structure and physical function. An example is spinal scoliosis (curvature of the spine), which is common in childhood-onset neuromuscular conditions. Clinical observation of spine flexibility is recommended until scoliosis is detected or until an individual is no longer able to walk. The degree of scoliosis can be accurately measured from an anteroposterior (front to back) spine X-ray and is referred to as the Cobb angle. Monitoring change in Cobb angle is essential, particularly prior to skeletal maturity. Published standards of care in Duchenne muscular dystrophy (Bushby et al. 2010; Birnkrant et al. 2018) and spinal muscular atrophy (Mercuri et al. 2018) dictate annual anterior-posterior spinal X-ray for individuals with a Cobb angle of 15° to 20° and every 6 months for those >20°.

FIELD TESTS

The most common tool used to measure joint range of motion objectively is a goniometer, as described in Chapter 2. Similarly, an inclinometer can be used to measure joint angles. The Charcot–Marie–Tooth disease Pediatric Scale mentioned in Table 9.2 uses an inclinometer (considered a tilt indicator as it measures angles or slopes with respect to gravity) to measure ankle flexibility in individuals with Charcot–Marie–Tooth disease as part test (part of the patient profile, rather than one of the test items per se) (Burns and The Inherited Neuropathies Consortium 2011). Inclinometers are more expensive than a goniometer, however, and whether they are more accurate than a goniometer is not known for measuring flexibility in childhood-onset neuromuscular conditions.

Effects of Physical Activity on the Flexibility of People With Childhood-Onset Neuromuscular Conditions

Natural history data in the Duchenne muscular dystrophy population supports the commonly held view that joint flexibility reduces with increasing age and thus likely with decreasing physical activity (Henricson et al. 2013). Increasing joint and muscle tightness has a negative impact on physical function, alters body mechanics, and can affect balance and the ability to stand, and a lack of flexibility in the legs has been shown to be related to the need for a wheelchair for mobility (McDonald et al. 1995).

PROMOTING A PHYSICALLY ACTIVE LIFESTYLE FOR PEOPLE WITH CHILDHOOD-ONSET NEUROMUSCULAR CONDITIONS

For children in the general population, inactivity (sedentary behaviour) contributes to muscle weakness and reduced flexibility (Carson et al. 2016) as well as pain (Baradaran Mahdavi et al. 2021) and reduced movement skills (Adank et al. 2018), all of which are primary health issues present in individuals with childhood-onset neuromuscular conditions. For people with neuromuscular conditions, being more physically activity also has benefits regarding weight management, reduction of the incidence of heart disease, osteoporosis, and diabetes (McDonald 2002). For individuals with Duchenne muscular dystrophy, some of the most commonly reported benefits across a variety of ages (and thus levels of physical ability) are those that support mental health, such as having fun, making friends, the thrill of winning, and reduced anxiety levels (Heutnick 2017). Therefore, to avoid the negative effects of inactivity and benefit from the positive effects of physical activity, promotion of a physically active lifestyle in this population is critical.

However, promoting a physically active lifestyle in people with childhood-onset neuromuscular conditions is not without its challenges. Fatigue (a feeling of exhaustion) is a common complaint for this group and could well be a barrier to physical activity engagement for at least some. For example, one study examining health-related qualify of life in a large group of males with Duchenne muscular dystrophy showed that the single biggest contributor to low quality of life was increasing levels of fatigue (Wei et al. 2016). Furthermore, with increasing age, males with Duchenne muscular dystrophy disengaged from participation in physical activity (Bendixen et al. 2012). In addition, when losing the ability to walk, males with Duchenne muscular dystrophy were less likely to be involved in physical activity than more established wheelchair users (De Valle et al. 2016). In addition to health issues, one of the most significant barriers to participation in physical activity by males with Duchenne muscular dystrophy is a lack of appropriate sporting facilities (Heutnick 2017). Other factors identified include a large distance from facilities, cost, and lack of time and interest in physical activity. Pain, lack of energy, and finding exercise 'too difficult' are also reported as significant barriers identified in other childhood-onset neuromuscular conditions (Phillips et al. 2009).

Given these challenges and barriers, the child- and family-centred approaches to addressing barriers and improving physical activity detailed in Chapter 5 should be considered when developing a physical activity programme for individuals with childhood-onset neuromuscular conditions, as should the training principles and precautions mentioned in this chapter for cardiorespiratory fitness and submaximal exercise capacity and muscular fitness. Any physical activity programme should be individualized and supervised, especially in the beginning, by a physical activity professional with expertise with the population.

REFERENCES

Adank AM, Van Kann DHH, Hoeboer JJAA, De Vries SI, Kremers SPJ, Vos SB (2018) Investigating motor competence in association with sedentary behavior and physical activity in 7- to 11-year-old children. *Int J Environ Res Public Health* **15**: 2470.

Bar-Or O (1996) Role of exercise in the assessment and management of neuromuscular disease in children. *Medicine and Science in Sports and Exercise* **28**: 421–427.

Baradaran Mahdavi S, Riahi R, Vahdatpour B, Kelishadi R (2021) Association between sedentary behavior and low back pain: a systematic review and meta-analysis. *Health Promot Perspect* **11**: 393–410.

Bartels B, Takken T, Blank AC, Van Moorsel H, Van der Pol WL, De Groot JF (2015) Cardiopulmonary exercise testing in children and adolescents with dystrophinopathies: a pilot study. *Pediatr Phys Ther* **27**: 227–234. **https://journals.lww.com/pedpt/Fulltext/2015/27030/Cardiopulmonary_Exercise_Testing_in_Children_and.4.aspx.**

Bendixen RM, Senesac C, Lott DJ, Vandenborne K (2012) Participation and quality of life in children with Duchenne muscular dystrophy using the International Classification of Functioning, Disability, and Health. *Health and Quality of Life Outcomes* **10**: 43.

Birnkrant DJ, Bushby K, Bann CM et al. (2018) Diagnosis and management of Duchenne muscular dystrophy, part 1: diagnosis, and neuromuscular, rehabilitation, endocrine, and gastrointestinal and nutritional management. *Lancet Neurol* **17**: 251–267.

Burns J, Ouvrier R, Estilow T et al. (2012) Validation of the Charcot–Marie–Tooth disease pediatric scale as an outcome measure of disability. *Annals of Neurology* **71**: 642–652.

Burns J, Sman AD, Cornett KMD et al. (2017) Safety and efficacy of progressive resistance exercise for Charcot–Marie–Tooth disease in children: a randomised, double-blind, sham-controlled trial. *Lancet Child Adolesc Health* **1**: 106–113.

Burns J, The Inherited Neuropathies Consortium (2011) *Charcot-Marie-Tooth Disease Pediatric Scale Equipment and Training Resource Kit* [online]. Available at: https://www.clinicaloutcomemeasures.org/calculators/cmtpeds/cmtpeds-training-and-resource-manual/ [Accessed 6 September 2022]. Note that the URL will first point to a registration page. After registering, the URL will point to the document.

Burns J, The Inherited Neuropathies Consortium (2022) *CMTPedS Calculator* [online]. Available at: https://www.clinicaloutcomemeasures.org/calculators/cmtpeds/ [Accessed 6 September 2022]. Note that the URL will first point to a registration page. After registering, the URL will point to the CMTPeds calculator.

Bushby K, Connor E (2011) Clinical outcome measures for trials in Duchenne muscular dystrophy: report from International Working Group meetings. *Clin Investig (Lond)* **1**: 1217–1235. **https://www.ncbi.nlm.nih.gov/pmc/articles/PMC3357954/pdf/nihms356627.pdf.**

Bushby K, Finkel R, Birnkrant DJ et al. (2010) Diagnosis and management of Duchenne muscular dystrophy, part 2: implementation of multidisciplinary care. *The Lancet Neurology* **9**: 177–189.

Carson V, Hunter S, Kuzik N et al. (2016) Systematic review of sedentary behaviour and health indicators in school-aged children and youth: an update. *Appl Physiol Nutr Metab* **41**: S240–S265.

Crisafulli S, Sultana J, Fontana A, Salvo F, Messina S, Trifiro G (2020) Global epidemiology of Duchenne muscular dystrophy: an updated systematic review and meta-analysis. *Orphanet J Rare Dis* **15**: 141.

Cup EH, Pieterse AJ, Ten Broek-Pastoor JM et al. (2007) Exercise therapy and other types of physical therapy for patients with neuromuscular diseases: a systematic review. *Archives of Physical Medicine and Rehabilitation* **88**: 1452–1464.

Darras BT (2015) *Neuromuscular Disorders of Infancy, Childhood, and Adolescence a Clinician's Approach*, 2nd ed. Amsterdam: Elsevier/Academic Press.

Davidson ZE, Truby H (2009) A review of nutrition in Duchenne muscular dystrophy. *J Hum Nutr Diet* **22**: 383–393.

De Lateur BJ, Giaconi RM (1979) Effect on maximal strength of submaximal exercise in Duchenne muscular dystrophy. *Am J Phys Med* **58**: 26–36.

De Valle KL, Davidson ZE, Kennedy RA, Ryan MM, Carroll KM (2016) Physical activity and the use of standard and complementary therapies in Duchenne and Becker muscular dystrophies. *Journal of Pediatric Rehabilitation Medicine* **9**: 55–63.

Dirks I, Koene S, Verbruggen R, Smeitink JA, Jansen M, Groot IJ (2016) Assisted 6-minute cycling test: an exploratory study in children. *Muscle Nerve* **54**: 232–238. **https://onlinelibrary.wiley.com/doi/10.1002/mus.25021** (the article is freely available on the Internet and can be located using a search engine).

Elliott SA, Davidson ZE, Davies PSW, Truby H (2015) A bedside measure of body composition in Duchenne muscular dystrophy. **52**: 82–87.

Florence J, Pandya S, King W et al. (1992) Intrarater reliability of manual muscle testing (medical research council scale) grades in Duchenne muscular dystrophy. *Physical Therapy* **72**: 115–122.

Florence JM, Fox PT, Planer GJ, Brooke MH (1985) Activity, creatine kinase, and myoglobin in Duchenne muscular dystrophy: a clue to etiology? *Neurology* **35**: 758–761.

Forrest G, Qian X (1999) Exercise in neuromuscular disease. *Neurorehabilitation* **13**: 135–139.

Glanzman A, O'Hagen M, McDermott MP et al. (2011) Validation of the Expanded Hammersmith Functional Motor Scale in Spinal Muscular Atrophy Type II and III. *Journal of Child Neurology* **26**: 1499–1507.

Hammer S, Toussaint M, Vollsaeter M et al. (2022) Exercise training in Duchenne muscular dystrophy: a systematic review and meta-analysis. *J Rehabil Med* **54**: jrm00250.

Hebert LJ, Maltais DB, Lepage C, Saulnier J, Crete M (2015) Hand-held dynamometry isometric torque reference values for children and adolescents. *Pediatr Phys Ther* **27**: 414–423. **https://www.ncbi.nlm.nih.gov/pmc/articles/PMC4581449/pdf/ppyty-27-414.pdf**.

Henricson EK, Abresch RT, Cnaan A et al. (2013) The cooperative international neuromuscular research group Duchenne natural history study: glucocorticoid treatment preserves clinically meaningful functional milestones and reduces rate of disease progression as measured by manual muscle testing and other commonly used clinical trial outcome measures. *Muscle Nerve* **48**: 55–67.

Heutnick L, Van Kampen N, Jansen M, De Groote IJM (2017) Physical activity in boys with Duchenne muscular dystrophy is lower and less demanding compared to healthy boys. *Journal of Child Neurology* **32**: 450–457.

Jansen M, De Jong M, Coes HM, Eggermont F, Van Alfen N, De Groot IJ (2012) The assisted 6-minute cycling test to assess endurance in children with a neuromuscular disorder. *Muscle Nerve* **46**: 520–530.

Jansen M, Van Alfen N, Geurts AC, De Groot IJ (2013) Assisted bicycle training delays functional deterioration in boys with Duchenne muscular dystrophy: the randomized controlled trial 'no use is disuse'. *Neurorehabil Neural Repair* **27**: 816–827.

Kilmer D (2002) Response to aerobic exercise training in humans with neuromuscular disease. *Am J Phys Med Rehabil* **81**(11 Suppl): S148–150.

Lott DJ, Taivassalo T, Cooke KD et al. (2021) Safety, feasibility, and efficacy of strengthening exercise in Duchenne muscular dystrophy. *Muscle Nerve* **63**: 320–326.

Markert CD, Case LE, Carter GT, Furlong PA, Grange RW (2012) Exercise and Duchenne muscular dystrophy: where we have been and where we need to go. *Muscle Nerve* **45**: 746–751.

Mayhew AG, Cano SJ, Scott E et al. (2013) Detecting meaningful change using the North Star Ambulatory Assessment in Duchenne muscular dystrophy. *Dev Med Child Neurol* **55**: 1046–1052. **https://onlinelibrary.wiley.com/doi/epdf/10.1111/dmcn.12220**.

Mayhew AG, Coratti G, Mazzone ES et al. (2020) Performance of upper limb module for Duchenne muscular dystrophy. *Dev Med Child Neurol* **62**: 633–639. For test directions and score sheet see the article's Appendix S1 at the following URL: **https://onlinelibrary.wiley.com/action/downloadSupplement?doi=10.1111%2Fdmcn.14361&file=dmcn14361-sup-0003-AppendixS1.pdf**. The article is freely available on the Internet and can be located using a search engine.

Mazzone E (2014) *Revised Upper Limb Module for SMA* [online]. Available at: **https://sjelden.no/course/2020-EMAN-funksjonsteser_spinraza/RULM-Generic-Manual-16-Dec-2014.pdf** [Accessed 31 August 2022].

Mazzone ES, Mayhew A, Montes J et al. (2017) Revised upper limb module for spinal muscular atrophy: development of a new module. *Muscle Nerve* **55**: 869–874. The Supplementary Fig. S1 is a scoring sheet for the Revised Upper Limb Module and can be found here: **https://onlinelibrary.wiley.com/action/downloadSupplement?doi=10.1002%2Fmus.25430&file=mus25430-sup-0001-suppinfo1.docx**. The article is freely available on the Internet and can be located using a search engine.

McDonald CM (2002) Physical activity, health impairments, and disability in neuromuscular disease. *Am J Phys Med Rehabil* **81**: S108–S120.

McDonald CM, Abresch RT, Carter GT et al. (1995) Profiles of neuromuscular diseases: Duchenne muscular dystrophy. *Am J Phys Med Rehabil* **74**: S70–92.

McDonald CM, Henricson EK, Abresch RT et al. (2013) The 6-minute walk test and other endpoints in Duchenne muscular dystrophy: longitudinal natural history observations over 48 weeks from a multicenter study. *Muscle Nerve* **48**: 343–356.

McDonald CM, Henricson EK, Han JJ et al. (2010) The 6-minute walk test as a new outcome measure in Duchenne muscular dystrophy. *Muscle Nerve* **41**: 500–510.

McPherson AC, Ball GD, Maltais DB et al. (2016) A call to action: setting the research agenda for addressing obesity and weight-related topics in children with physical disabilities. *Child Obes* **12**: 59–69.

Mercuri E, Coratti G, Messina S et al. (2016) Revised North Star Ambulatory Assessment for young boys with Duchenne muscular dystrophy. *PLoS One* **11**: e0160195.

Mercuri E, Finkel RS, Muntoni F et al. (2018) Diagnosis and management of spinal muscular atrophy: Part 1: Recommendations for diagnosis, rehabilitation, orthopedic and nutritional care. *Neuromuscul Disord* **28**: 103–115.

Merlini L, Dell'Accio D, Granata C (1995) Reliability of dynamic strength knee muscle testing in children. *Journal of Orthopaedic & Sports Physical Therapy* **22**: 73–76.

Merlini L, Mazzone ES, Solari A, Morandi L (2002) Reliability of hand-held dynamometry in spinal muscular atrophy. *Muscle & Nerve* **26**: 64–70.

Montes J, McDermott MP, Martens WB et al. (2010) Six-Minute Walk Test demonstrates motor fatigue in spinal muscular atrophy. *Neurology* **74**: 833–838.

Moore GE, Lindenmayer AW, McConchie GA, Ryan MM, Davidson ZE (2016) Describing nutrition in spinal muscular atrophy: a systematic review. *Neuromuscul Disord* **26**: 395–404.

Phillips M, Flemming N, Tsintzas K (2009) An exploratory study of physical activity and perceived barriers to exercise in ambulant people with neuromuscular disease compared with unaffected controls. *Clinical Rehabil* **23**: 746–755.

Ramsey D, Scoto M, Mayhew A et al. (2017) Revised Hammersmith Scale for spinal muscular atrophy: a SMA specific clinical outcome assessment tool. *PLoS One* **12**: e0172346. For test directions and score sheet see the article's Appendix S1 at the following URL: **https://doi.org/10.1371/journal.pone.0172346.s001**.

Ricotti V, Ridout DA, Pane M et al. (2016) The NorthStar Ambulatory Assessment in Duchenne muscular dystrophy: considerations for the design of clinical trials. *J Neurol Neurosurg Psychiatry* **87**: 149–155.

Scott E, Eagle M, Mayhew A et al. (2012) Development of a functional assessment scale for ambulatory boys with Duchenne muscular dystrophy. *Physiother Res Int* **17**: 101–109.

Smartnet, PNCR (2009) *Expanded Hammersmith Functional Motor Scale for SMA (HFMSE)* [online]. Available at: https://www.fundame.net/documentacion/Hammersmith%20Functional%20Motor%20Scale%20Expanded%20for%20SMA%20Type%20II%20and%20III%20-%20Manual%20of%20Procedures.pdf [Accessed 6 September 2022].

UK North Star Clinical Network (2017) *North Star Ambulatory Assessment (NSAA)* [online]. Available at: https://www.musculardystrophyuk.org/static/s3fs-public/2021-08/NSAA%20_Manual_%2015102020.pdf?VersionId=BaPGDWk5TxA3rtF2DDipAVYlOJ5Eoumo [Accessed 6 September 2022].

Utter AC, Robertson RJ, Nieman DC, Kang J (2002) Children's OMNI Scale of Perceived Exertion: walking/running evaluation. *Med Sci Sports Exerc* **34**: 139–144. **https://journals.lww.com/acsm-msse/Fulltext/2002/01000/Children_s_OMNI_Scale_of_Perceived_Exertion_.21.aspx**.

Van Mil E, Schoeber N, Calvert RE, Bar-Or O (1996) Optimization of force in the Wingate Test for children with a neuromuscular disease. *Med Sci Sports Exerc* **28**: 1087–1092.

Voet NBM (2019) Exercise in neuromuscular disorders: a promising intervention. *Acta Myol* **38**: 207–214.

Voet NBM, Van der Kooi EL, Riphagen II, Lindeman E, Van Engelen BGM, Geurts ACH (2010) Strength training and aerobic exercise training for muscle disease. *Cochrane Database of Systematic Reviews* (1): CD003907.

Wei Y, Speechley K, Zou G, Cambell C (2016) Factors associated with Health related quality of life in children with Duchenne muscular dystrophy. *Journal of Child Neurology* **31**: 879–886.

White CM, Pritchard J, Turner-Stokes L (2004) Exercise for people with peripheral neuropathy. *Cochrane Database of Systematic Reviews* (4): CD003904.

White CM, Van Doorn PA, Garssen MP, Stockley RC (2014) Interventions for fatigue in peripheral neuropathy. *Cochrane Database of Systematic Reviews* **12**: CD008146.

CHAPTER 10

Intellectual Disability

*Anne-Stine Dolva, Roald Undlien, Kaja Giltvedt,
and Andreas T Sandfossen*

What are the keys to fitness and physical activity for individuals with intellectual disability? 'An extra push and extra support' was a simple answer from one of the parents interviewed for the purpose of this chapter. In this chapter, we will provide some essential information to help better understand this quote.

This chapter begins with an overview of intellectual disability, including diagnostic criteria, common impairments, comorbidities, and medications. Specific diagnoses characterized with intellectual disability are also mentioned. This is followed by a review of the health-related fitness components of cardiorespiratory fitness and submaximal exercise capacity, muscular fitness, body composition, and flexibility. These terms are defined in Chapter 2. For each component, information is provided on why and how to evaluate it, and either intellectual disability-specific adaptation principles (cardiorespiratory fitness and submaximal exercise capacity, muscular fitness) or a discussion about how physical activity affects the component (body composition, flexibility). The chapter ends with an overview of guidelines on how to promote a physically active lifestyle for people with intellectual disability exemplified by stories of lived experience.

Health-related fitness tests are classified as laboratory or field tests. Laboratory tests are often employed in research or specialized clinical contexts, while field tests are used in both research, clinical, and community settings. Chapter 2 provides a more detailed description of both these types of tests. General safety considerations are provided in Chapter 3, and general training principles and motivational factors are presented in Chapters 4 and 5.

WHAT IS INTELLECTUAL DISABILITY?

Intellectual disability (intellectual developmental disorder) is characterized as 'a significantly reduced ability to understand new or complex information and to learn and apply new skills (impaired intelligence)' (World Health Organization 2016). It originates before the age of 18 years, has a lasting effect on development, and affects an individual's ability to cope independently. Diagnostic criteria for intellectual disability emphasize both cognitive capacity (IQ) and adaptive functioning, resulting in the need for extraordinary supports for a person to participate in activities. Adaptive functioning is what a person typically does in their environment (what some people call 'performance'), rather than what the person may be capable of doing (what some people call 'capacity'). There are numerous causes of intellectual disability and great variation among individuals. Intellectual disability includes a broad range of mental impairments, and synonymous terms include cognitive disability, developmental delay, and learning disability.

For many years, individuals with intellectual disability have been considered a homogeneous group. Advances in genetics and development, however, have improved the understanding of intellectual disabilities and atypical development over the life span (Hodapp and Fidler 1999). Individuals with various genetic syndromes have shown atypical neurodevelopment leading to some areas of functioning that are severely affected and other areas that are less so (Karmiloff-Smith 1998). Thus, in order to provide optimal support and create opportunities one needs to understand what makes it easy or hard for an individual to become, and to stay, physically active. This understanding is dependent both on an individual's impairments or health condition and the extent to which environmental factors support the individual's participation.

In this chapter, we will apply intellectual disability as the general term, referring to the wide range of limitations in intellectual functioning and adaptive behaviour. In addition, we will use knowledge related to the diagnosis of Down syndrome, Prader–Willi syndrome, and Williams syndrome with the aim of highlighting some population-specific issues associated with health-related fitness and physical activity. Therefore, a brief introduction to the three chromosomal disorder diagnosis is provided.

Down syndrome is the most common cause of intellectual disability, caused by issues related to a third chromosome 21, affecting approximately 1:700/900 live births per year (Roizen and Patterson 2003). Most individuals with Down syndrome have a mild to moderate intellectual disability (Hodapp, Evans, and Gray 1999). Williams syndrome is a chromosome disorder (chromosome 7), affecting proximately 1:10 000 (Strømme, Bjørnstad, and Ramstad 2002). Children with Williams syndrome have characteristic facial features, mild to moderate intellectual disability, and an extroverted personality (Morris 2013). Prader–Willi syndrome is a rare congenital condition caused by issues related to chromosome 15, resulting in mild to moderate intellectual disability. Children with Prader–Willi syndrome have a characteristic increased interest in food resulting in overweight and obesity, and they have difficulties with social skills (Lukosh et al. 2014). The prevalence is reported to be about 1:25.000 (Vogels et al. 2004).

COMMON IMPAIRMENTS AND COMORBIDITIES

For people with intellectual disability, impairments in the central nervous system (CNS) result in limitations in intellectual functioning. Intellectual functioning refers to reasoning, planning, problem solving, abstract thinking, comprehending complex ideas, learning quickly, and learning from experience (Schalock et al. 2010). The causes and aetiology of impaired intellectual functioning are many and varied, as is the range and type of CNS impairments. In addition, CNS impairments may predispose to other specific health problems or medical conditions.

Specific conditions are seen with chromosome disorders. One example is with Williams syndrome. The deficiency on chromosome 7 is associated with, among other things, decreased elasticity of tissues influencing joints' range of motion. Due to this, contractures of knees and ankle joints may develop in early childhood. Literature suggests that physical activity and exercise for joint range of motion may help to prevent contractures, and development of type 2 diabetes with Williams syndrome (Morris 2013).

More commonly, the health status of persons with intellectual disability changes with advancing age and is often accompanied by impairments related to vision and hearing, mobility, comorbid mental illness, and, for some, also challenging behaviour. For more general information, see Chapter 3.

COMMON MEDICATIONS

In general, intellectual disability is associated with an increased risk for health problems, and differences among individuals vary greatly. There are no common medications used by people with intellectual disability, rather medication use depends on individual health conditions. Medications for syndrome-specific conditions are well known, for example those related to hypothyroidism in Down syndrome, a growth hormone deficit in Prader–Willi syndrome, and with cardiovascular abnormalities in Williams syndrome.

Chapter 3 provides an overview of safety considerations that clinicians should be aware of in light of the impairments and other health issues that people in this group may have.

CARDIORESPIRATORY FITNESS

Cardiorespiratory fitness levels are low across the entire population with intellectual disability beginning in childhood, with further decline with increasing age (Oppewal et al. 2013). Furthermore, females have lower cardiorespiratory fitness levels than males. In general, physical inactivity is likely to contribute to low cardiorespiratory fitness levels.

Testing

The tests described in Chapter 4 are for the most part feasible for individuals with intellectual disability, as long as they have sufficient motor skills to perform the test and cognitive skills to follow test instructions. It is usually helpful, however, to practise the test before the actual measurements are taken and to ensure that the individual feels comfortable with all the steps. That may include, for example, practising riding the exercise bicycle or walking and running on the treadmill and wearing the mouth piece or mask for measuring peak oxygen uptake.

Training

The general principles for exercise training to improve cardiorespiratory fitness, outlined in Chapter 2, apply to this population. The suggestions for less fit individuals are particularly relevant.

MUSCULAR FITNESS

One condition often associated with intellectual disability is hypotonia, which known to co-occur with Prader–Willi syndrome, Williams syndrome, and Down syndrome. Hypotonia is the most common terminology used to describe decreased muscular tone and is commonly accompanied with hypermobility of joints (O'Sullivan 2007). Low muscle tone may not be directly related to low muscle strength or endurance. However, literature suggests that hypotonia and generalized muscle weakness are correlated, even though this is not universally accepted (Martin et al. 2005).

Testing

Given the level of motor skill and cooperation required for strength testing, it is crucial that these tests are practised before the actual measurements are taken. Trial and error may be needed to find the most appropriate tests for a given individual.

Training

Muscle strength and anaerobic fitness are lower in children and adolescents with intellectual disability than in peers without disabilities (Guerra, Giné-Garriga, and Fernhall 2009; Samuel, Saxena, and Aranha 2016). The general principles for exercise training to improve muscular fitness as noted in Chapter 2 apply to this population. The suggestions for beginners are particularly relevant.

BODY COMPOSITION

There is a high prevalence of obesity and obesity-related secondary conditions in people with intellectual disability. Needless to say, obesity often leads to different negative health conditions, such as hypertension, diabetes, arthritis, stroke, stress, depression, and respiratory diseases (Poirier et al. 2006; Krokstad, Knudtsen, and Hunt 2011). In addition, children with obesity generally experience stigmatization (Latner and Stunkard 2003). Children and adolescents with Down syndrome, Prader–Willi syndrome, as well as autism spectrum disorder (see Chapter 12) are found to have an increased risk for obesity and overweight due to a variety of physiological mechanisms and behavioural tendencies (Murray and Ryan-Krause 2010; Nordstrøm 2015).

Obesity with Prader–Willi syndrome is typical, as newborn infants show feeding problems with a failure to thrive and must generally be tube-fed for a short time. However, children with Prader–Willi syndrome show an increased interest in food that is frequently associated with obesity. Typically they do not experience a feeling of satiety, even after a big meal, due to abnormal hypothalamic function (Vogels et al. 2004). Thus, a relatively strict diet with a fixed amount of food for meals to reduce calorie intake, combined with regular physical activity, is important. Children with Prader–Willi syndrome who are treated with growth hormones may have an increased muscle mass and linear growth (Emerick and Vogt 2013).

An opposite challenge to obesity is seen in children with Williams syndrome. For those children reduced absorbency, vomiting, and colic due to hypercalcemia (high levels of calcium) is common. Treatment involves a diet of foods with reduced levels of calcium and vitamin D, and a recommended gradual increase up to normal intake (Morris et al. 1988). Transitioning to solid foods takes time and difficulties with nutrition often continue in early childhood. It is important to ensure good nutrition if someone in this situation is going to increase their level of physical activity.

Testing

The body composition tests mentioned in Chapter 2 are for the most part appropriate for individuals with intellectual disability. However, if obesity or underweight is a severe problem the more precise laboratory-based assessments may be the preferred tests.

Training

The strength capacity of children and adolescents with intellectual disability is low compared with their peers without disabilities (González-Agüero et al. 2010). The general principles for exercise training to improve body composition noted in Chapter 4 apply to those with intellectual disability.

FLEXIBILITY

Hypotonia and increased laxity of joints may lead to abnormal compensatory postures to achieve stability (Morris 2013). With age, individuals may develop a stereotypical gait pattern due to hypotonicity of specific lower extremity muscles. For example, children with Williams syndrome may develop contractures of the knee and ankle joint already in early childhood, but still develop adequate functional abilities to perform a variety of physical activities.

Testing and Training

The flexibility tests mentioned in Chapter 4 are appropriate for individuals with intellectual disability, as are the general principles for improving flexibility where it is warranted.

PROMOTING A PHYSICALLY ACTIVE LIFESTYLE IN PERSONS WITH INTELLECTUAL DISABILITY

Systematic measurement of physical activity with individuals with intellectual disability is limited. A systematic review conducted by Hinckson and Curtis (2013) found that accelerometers and pedometers are mainly used, and heart rate telemetry is less used because children with intellectual disability often refuse to wear such monitors. Subjective measures of physical activity are also used, including questionnaires, activity logs, and interviews with parents. However, knowledge is limited regarding frequency, intensity, and duration measures of physical activity with young people with intellectual disability (Frey, Stanish, and Temple 2008). Furthermore, a pilot study conducted in 2009 showed that people with intellectual disability can be highly trustworthy informers when describing their own level of physical activity (Ingebrigtsen and Aspvik 2009). The study showed a strong correlation between self-reported effort through questionnaires and the actual physical activity measured with accelerometers. See Chapter 4 for principles for measuring physical activity.

As for all individuals at all ages, physical activity improves fitness, functional ability, growth, cultural awareness, and psychological well-being, and helps establish relationships in the community (Murphy and Carbone 2008). In addition, physical activity and fitness are found to reduce the risk of, for example, diabetes and cardiovascular disease (World Health Organization 2010).

Like all people, individuals with intellectual disability benefit from being physically active (Bartlo and Klein 2011), and physical activity is the single most effective way to improve health (Robertson et al. 2000). Within the limitations of measuring physical activity in this group, a broad mass of research suggests that individuals with intellectual disability are far more likely to live a sedentary life and engage less in physical activity than their peers for various reasons (Esposito et al. 2012; Nordstrøm 2015). The reasons for this appear complex. Individual differences in the degree of engagement in physical activity are significant, based on the extent (mild to profound) of intellectual disability (Bartlo and Klein 2011). General low individual motivation for physical activity has also been described (Kosma, Cardinal, and Rintala 2002), and many people with intellectual disability seem to prefer sedentary activities (Esposito et al. 2012).

While intellectual disability manifests primarily as limitations in intellectual functioning, the capacity to participate in activities is also influenced. Intellectual disability is not defined by the impairments itself but by the person's functioning. This can be described as a mismatch between the person's capacity and the activity and participation expectations of the context. The person–environment fit model of intellectual disability leads to the need to emphasize support needs. Thus, individual support may be crucial to enable a child or adult to participate successfully in the settings and activities of their environment. The quote from one of our parents points directly to this: 'Extra push and extra support'. What the extra push and extra support involves, however, will vary among individuals and their support needs. Nevertheless, more information is needed to better understand the relationship between the individual and their environmental opportunities for being physically active.

Motivation and Support

In the following section we describe some general supports or strategies that may increase individual functioning and/or adapt the environment or physical activities to enhance participation in physical activity. Motivation and support may enhance the chance for many people with intellectual disability to participate in physical activity. Finding out what the child wants to do is key to maintaining motivation.

Individuals with Down syndrome tend to have low motivation for physical activity (Kosma et al. 2002). Enjoyable and even unstructured physical activity is found to enhance motivation and engagement (Downs et al. 2013, 2014). Identifying personal interest and motivation for physical activity is important, as is giving choices for activities to pursue. Opportunities to choose activities freely has been described to facilitate participation (Brown, O'Keefe, and Stagnitti 2011), even if support is required to make a choice (Mahy et al. 2010). Supporting individual wishes and qualifications is also known to enable individuals with intellectual disability to function in typical life situations

(Thompson et al. 2009). Thus, having fun seems to motivate, and the doing itself is important. Social participation and being involved in a peer group for physical activity are also motivating (Kollstad, Dolva, and Kleiven 2015). In addition, music has been described as an important motivational factor for individuals with Williams syndrome to be physically active (Dykens et al. 2005).

Parents who initiate and engage in physical activity themselves also facilitate their children to be active (Menear 2007; Barr and Shields 2011). Moreover, the support from parents in choosing activities, providing support, and using their knowledge of what their children need to do to get fit are also found to influence successful physical activity participation (Dolva, Kleiven, and Kollstad 2014).

In sports programmes, support or help from peers or other attendants outside the family is also found to influence individuals in a positive way (Hutzler and Korsensky 2010). Several studies have also noted the importance of the social roles of assistants and other supportive people. In Norway, a specific method *Fritid med bistand* [Leisure with support] (Midtsundstad 2013), using competent assistants, is based on the principles of empowerment. The method has proved successful in providing individualized support to persons with intellectual disability in physical activity.

Routines in activity programmes may be important. For some persons with Prader–Willi syndrome with rigid behaviour, changing routines in a programme can cause stress and dropout. Unchanged routines throughout physical activity programmes may avoid such dropouts (e.g. Castner et al. 2014).

ALLSPORT GROUP IN A NORWEGIAN CONTEXT

To better understand what 'extra push and extra support' looks like in practice, we provide an example of a successful physical activity programme, 'AllSport'. We interviewed six young participants of the AllSport programme and obtained the experiences of some of their parents.

In Norway, ordinary sports federations organize all types of sports, including for individuals with disabilities. We will briefly describe one such sports activity called 'Nordstrand AllSport group for children and youth with intellectual disability'. This group provides activities, such as AllSport-basic, handball, football, swimming, and golf. The Nordstrand AllSport group was started in 2000 in Oslo, and it currently involves 70 members with various disabilities, aged 5 to 20 years. The organizing concepts build upon the philosophy and principals of the 'F-words in childhood disability': function, family, fitness, fun, friends, and future (Rosenbaum and Gorter 2011).

Most of the participants in the group still live with their parents, and the parents organize everything from being in place at the right time, or being there at all, to ensuring the participants are wearing appropriate outfits. In the transition from youth to adulthood challenges may arise, especially when it comes to organizing and maintaining participation in the 'AllSport' group. It is important that all children with disabilities get the chance to start out early with facilitated practice, so that they get the same chances as all other children to be physically active. By offering a variety of experiences through sports, the participants may achieve better health and healthy growth as they develop towards adulthood. Challenges ahead will include getting providers to take responsibilities from the parents to help the young adults continue to be physically active.

Other important aspects of organizing this kind of AllSport group are that the coaches have the opportunity to learn about intellectual disability, that they have knowledge about the sports they teach, and that they try to follow the philosophy and principals of the 'F-words' (Rosenbaum and Gorter 2011).

PARTICIPANT EXPERIENCES

Six participant of the 'AllSports' group, aged 10 to 21 years, took part in a group interview to share their experiences about fitness and physical activity. There were four females and two males, and they had Down syndrome, Prader–Willi syndrome, or Williams syndrome. They were asked to come with their parents and bring with them three photos of sports and physical activity that they were particularly fond of. They were asked to talk about the pictures, say something about why they exercise and why it is important for them to be physically active either through organized sports or through everyday activities. Parents were present in order to supplement and support their children with the interview. The interview was taped and transcribed, and analysed with simple content analysis, displaying three themes.

Variation in Activities

One by one the young people talked about their favourite activities in the photos. The activities listed were running and the AllSport group, handball, jumping on the trampoline, playing Wii, organized dancing, and competitive gymnastics. After the interview there was a follow-up exchange of experience. On the follow-up exchange of experience they showed pictures and talked about cycling, skiing, horseback riding, swimming/pool activities, football, floorball, golf, and hiking, for example in the mountains. All mentioned several activities they liked to do do (Figures 10.1, 10.2, and 10.3).

Sports and Activity as an Important Social Arena

Talking about the pictures, almost everyone spontaneously mentioned that meeting and being with friends was what they liked the most about the activities. As one female said: 'I prefer to run with friends, and then to concentrate on running.' This was also

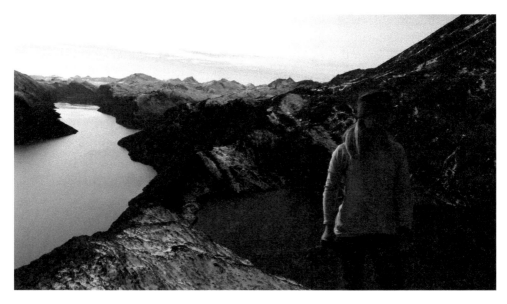

Figure 10.1 Mountain tracking: Besseggen, Norway

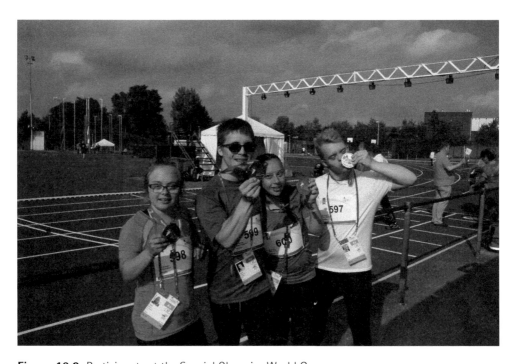

Figure 10.2 Participants at the Special Olympics World Games

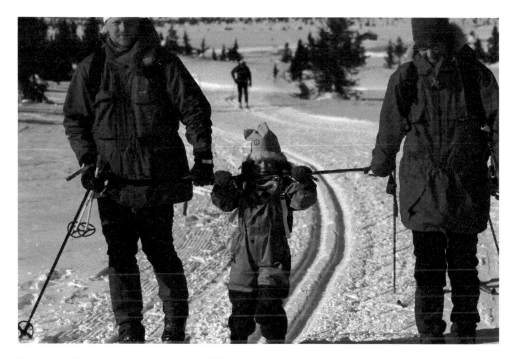

Figure 10.3 Learning cross-country skiing

supported by her parents: 'Meeting friends is an important motivator for taking part in sports.' Furthermore, one of the males said that when he attends handball he also meets with his girlfriend. This was also emphasized by several others, when talking about meeting their boyfriend or girlfriend at different physical activities. One female even talked about when she had a 'trampoline-date': 'We jumped, I think I jumped on the trampoline for almost an hour with my boyfriend. It was the best!' Her parents added that this is a very nice way to motivate for physical activity: 'We organize, for example, ski dates, bike dates, and ice skating dates. We see that this is a very nice way to spend time with both boyfriends/girlfriends and other friends.'

Fitness and Emotions

Talking about their physical activities, the interviewer tried to challenge the young people to talk both about their likes and dislikes. One said that he knows why he feels happy when he plays floorball: 'It is because I know that my team will win.' Another said that he gets really angry and swears when he gets tackled or loses the ball during a handball match. Several of the young people said that they got very upset when they lost a game. One of the young people had participated in gymnastics in the Special Olympics World Games. She talked about how brilliant she was and that she won the whole competition. Her mother clarified and said: 'You won at least over yourself.' She also reported that her daughter trained four times a week and 2 to 3 hours each time, in preparation for the World Championship: 'You were able to do this because you thought it was fun,' the mother said. Several of the participants expressed that they liked to compete and win, exemplified by the following quote: 'To participate in the 400m run, I have to practise a lot. I like that. I love to run and win.'

Why Is Fitness Important?

At the end of the interview, the topic 'Why is fitness important?' was discussed. One participant said that it is important to practise a lot to score goals: 'Yes you need to exercise plenty to get some more muscles and to be fast and to score.' One participant claimed that if you do not train hard, you have to be better and smoother, and keep on, until you get very fit and strong. One mother said that her daughter often got scared because she thought that her heart could jump out of her body because it pounded so hard and fast. One of the others answered: 'I think I need to run over and over again, so that I can bear to run constantly. My wish is to be able to run to the North Pole!' One of the females also started a discussion with her father that she wanted to start gymnastics classes for children with low muscle mass because she needed it, and she had a friend who attended this type of class.

The most important factors for these six young people to engage in sports and physical activities seemed to be being with and meeting friends. To some, competing and winning were also very important.

PARENTAL EXPERIENCES

For the purpose of this chapter, a group interview was conducted with a strategic sample of the parents of the five adolescents with intellectual disability. The parents who agreed to participate were all employed full-time, with above average education and income. We asked the parents about their experiences with fitness and physical activity with their son or daughter. The interview was taped, transcribed, and analysed with content analysis, displaying three main themes: the parental role, parental strategies, and future worries.

The Parental Role

The parents agreed that their role in actively facilitating fitness and physical activity from early childhood was of considerable importance for a healthy life for their children. The specific syndrome the child had was irrelevant, as the challenges posed to each were the same. It did not matter if it was Down syndrome or Prader–Willi syndrome: their aim was to establish a habitual physically active lifestyle for their child. To succeed with this, they used their engagement, initiative, and leisure time. This finding is consistent with a 'non-categorical' approach to childhood disability (Pless and Pinkerton 1975).

First, they worked to include fitness and physical activity in their everyday family life. In addition to physical family activities, they valued organized activities. As adolescents, they mainly participated in organized physical activities adapted for individuals with intellectual disabilities. In addition, a few of them had participated in ordinary organized physical activities during their childhood.

Parents were aware that where they lived provided different opportunities for adapted organized activities. Some living in urban areas experienced the privilege of choosing from a range of different sports. Some told how they, together with other parents, had initiated sports for children with intellectual disability. As with most parents, they were drivers to and from activities. Safety challenges in relation to urban traffic are well known issues for people with intellectual disabilities, and the parents were aware that their driver role could be long lasting.

Parents experienced that 'these children with syndromes need an extra push and extra support' to get fit and physically active. One of the parents verbalized general advice on behalf of the group: 'It is important to drop restricted thinking. They do have the same possibilities as most others; it is just some adaptations are needed.' The parents placed great importance on focusing on the possibilities rather than the limitations, and to some degree, 'try for yourself instead of blindly trusting advices for what your child can and cannot do'.

Several of the parents strived to balance leisure time in the family and between family members, as 'It is thanks to the parental effort that she is active'.

Parental Strategies

Motivation and facilitating participation in physical activity was a great issue for the group, and they often used different strategies. As one of the parents clarified: 'Despite having the same syndrome, no one of them are alike.' Thus, strategies were different for each individual, while many issues were shared by most parents.

From early childhood, parents were used to facilitating participation in physical activities without questioning their role. A straightforward way was saying 'Here we go!' and not giving any real option whether to come or not. Even today, their adolescents accept it. This did not mean that their children were forced to participate in activities. One of the parents presented a basic philosophy: 'They love to be challenged within their range of mastery.' It seemed to reflect that parents participated in choosing suitable activities, based on knowledge about their child's preferences and skills. For example, some loved to compete and participated in the Special Olympics World Games, managing the rules of sports, and loved football or handball. Some were happy to join with others and participated in general AllSports. However, individual differences are present, as with all young people.

Another strategy well known and much used by the parents was food restrictions. In their experience, the association of food with all kinds of celebrations, social gatherings, and parties challenged the fitness levels of their children with intellectual disability. As a response to this, one family applied the following strategy: 'We have two hotdogs and one piece of cake as a limit.' They admitted that it could be hard for their son to remember this rule, but mostly it worked.

The parents also thought that their adolescents would rarely be 'self-driven' in relation to physical activity. As many of them only met with friends and other adolescents during organized physical activity, this became a strong motivator to socialize. One parent expressed: 'Physical activity is fun, because that's where friends are.' Another parent added: 'It is only being with friends that is beating the computer.'

Parental Future Worries Related to a Lifelong Healthy Lifestyle

As seen above, fitness and physical activity for people with intellectual disabilities are in most ways the same as for all young people. Still, parents find their proactive role and strategies of considerable importance. As long as their children live at home, fitness and physical activity are mainly under control. For a more general overview of how to promote a physically active lifestyle, see Chapter 5.

A future worry for the parents was related to the time when their adolescents will move into their own or shared apartments with assistance in daily life. Many parents observed that young adults gained a lot of weight during the first years out of the family home. Parents were critical of how waffles and pizza seemed to be prioritized rather than healthy nutrition and physical activity. They claimed that there is a lack of competence in nutrition and physical activity for the assistants, and questioned whether these issues were emphasized within their education. In addition, some parents disagreed on focusing on self-determination in issues like food and physical activity, and questioned why habits and rules learned earlier in life could not be used. One parent commented: 'With junk food and low physical activity they are destroying their adulthood.'

SUMMARY

The quote from a parent, 'extra push and extra support' has been a common thread throughout this chapter. The quote exposed both knowledge and experience. What the extra push and extra support involve, however, will vary among individuals and their support needs. Yet, it must be based on identifying the misfit between an individual's capacity and the activity and participation expectations of the context. As we have seen, the person–environment fit model of intellectual disability leads to the need to emphasize support and support needs. Therefore, promoting a physically active lifestyle in intellectual disability must be individualized and the 'push and support' should be adapted to the individual. Finally, with the voice of the children and young people themselves, what matters most in promoting a physically active lifestyle is being with friends and having fun. It is of great importance that interventions start at an early age, making physical activity a family issue and part of an active lifestyle. In doing so, it becomes part of daily life rather than an 'add-on' that has to be done.

REFERENCES

Barr M, Shields N (2011) Identifying the barriers and facilitators to participation in physical activity for children with Down syndrome. *Journal of Intellectual Disability Research* **55**: 1020–1033. 10.1111/j.1365-2788.2011.01425.x.

Bartlo P, Klein PJ (2011) Physical activity benefits and needs in adults with intellectual disabilities: systematic review of the literature. *American Journal of Intellectual and Developmental Disabilities* **116**: 220–232.

Brown T, O'Keefe S, Stagnitti K (2011) Activity preferences and participation of school-age children living in urban and rural environments. *Occupational Therapy in Health Care* **25**: 225–239.

Castner DM, Tucker JM, Wilson KS, Rubin DA (2014) Patterns of habitual physical activity in youth with and without Prader-Willi syndrome. *Research in Developmental Disabilities* **35**: 3081–3088.

Dolva A-S, Kleiven J, Kollstad M (2014) Actual leisure of Norwegian adolescents with Down syndrome. *Journal of Intellectual Disabilities* **18**: 159–175.

Downs SJ, Boddy LM, Knowles ZR, Fairclough SJ, Stratton G (2013) Exploring opportunities available and perceived barriers to physical activity engagement in children and young people with Down syndrome. *European Journal of Special Needs Education* **28**: 270–287. 10.1080/08856257.2013.768453.

Downs SJ, Knowles ZR, Fairclough SJ et al. (2014) Exploring teachers' perceptions on physical activity engagement for children and young people with intellectual disabilities. *European Journal of Special Needs Education* **29**: 402–414. 10.1080/08856257.2014.906979

Dykens EM, Rosner BA, Ly T, Smith J (2005) Music and anxiety in Williams syndrome: a harmonious or discordant relationship? *American Journal on Mental Retardation* **110**: 346–358.

Emerick JE, Vogt KS (2013) Endocrine manifestations and management of Prader-Willi syndrome. *International Journal of Pediatric Endocrinology* **2013**: 14. 10.1186/1687-9856-2013-14.

Esposito PE, MacDonald M, Hornyak JE, Ulrich DA (2012) Physical activity patterns of youth with Down syndrome. *Intellectual and Developmental Disabilities* **50**: 109–119.

Frey GC, Stanish HI, Temple VA (2008) Physical activity of youth with intellectual disability: review and research agenda. *Adapted Physical Avtivity Quarterly* **25**: 95–117.

González-Agüero A, Vicente-Rodríguez G, Moreno L, Guerra-Balic M, Ara I, Casajus J (2010) Health-related physical fitness in children and adolescents with Down syndrome and response to training. *Scandinavian Journal of Medicine & Science in Sports* **20**: 716–724.

Guerra M, Giné-Garriga M, Fernhall B (2009) Reliability of Wingate testing in adolescents with Down syndrome. *Pediatric Exercise Science* **21**: 47–54.

Hinckson EA, Curtis A (2013) Measuring physical activity in children and youth living with intellectual disabilities: a systematic review. *Res Dev Disabil* **34**: 72–86.

Hodapp RM, Evans DW, Gray FL (1999) Intellectual development in children with Down syndrome. In: Rondal JA, Perera J, Nadel L, editors, *Down Syndrome: A Review of Current Knowledge*. London: Whurr Publishers, pp 124–132.

Hodapp RM, Fidler DJ (1999) Special education and genetics: connections for the 21st century. *Journal of Special Education* **33**: 130–137.

Hutzler Y, Korsensky O (2010) Motivational correlates of physical activity in persons with an intellectual disability: a systematic literature review. *Journal of Intellectual Disability Research* **54**: 767–786. 10.1111/j.1365-2788.2010.01313.x.

Ingebrigtsen JE, Aspvik NP (2009) Fysisk aktivitet og idrett: en pilotstudie av utviklingshemmedes fysiske aktivitet. *NTNU Samfunnsforskning AS, Senter for idrettsforskning*.

Karmiloff-Smith A (1998) Development itself is the key to understand developmental disorders. *Trends in Cognitive Science* **2**: 289–398.

Kollstad M, Dolva A-S, Kleiven J (2015) Independent and supported physical leisure activities of adoelscents with Down syndrome. *Ergoterapeuten* **58**: 38–47.

Kosma M, Cardinal BJ, Rintala P (2002) Motivating individuals with disabilities to be physically active. *Quest* **54**: 116–132.

Krokstad S, Knudtsen MS, HUNT (2011) *Folkehelse i endring: Helseundersøkelsen Nord-Trøndelag: HUNT 1 (1984–86) – HUNT 2 (1995–97) – HUNT 3 (2006–08) = Public health development: The HUNT study, Norway: HUNT 1 (1984–86) – HUNT 2 (1995–97) – HUNT 3 (2006–08) Public health development The HUNT study, Norway: HUNT 1 (1984–86) – HUNT 2 (1995–97) – HUNT 3 (2006–08)*.

Latner JD, Stunkard AJ (2003) Getting worse: the stigmatization of obese children. *Obesity* **11**: 452–456.

Lukosh A, Hokken-Koelega AC, van der Lugt A, White T (2014) Reduced cortical complexity in children with Prader-Willi syndrome and its association with cognitive impairment and developmental delay. *PloS One* **9**: e107320.

Mahy J, Shields N, Taylor NF, Dodd KJ (2010) Identifying facilitators and barriers to physical activity for adults with Down syndrome. *Journal of Intellectual Disability Research* **54**: 795–805. 10.1111/j.1365-2788.2010.01308.x.

Martin K, Inman J, Kirschner A, Deming K, Gumber R, Voelkner L (2005) Characteristic of hypotonia in children: a consensus opinion of pediatric occupational and physical therapists. *Pediatric Physical Therapy* **17**: 275–282.

Menear KS (2007) Parents' perceptions of health and physical activity needs of children with Down syndrome. *Down Syndrome Research and Practice* **12**: 60–68.

Midtsundstad A (2013) *Fritid med bistand [Leisure With Support]*. Bergen: Fagbokforlaget.

Morris CA (2013) Williams syndrome. *GeneReviews* [online]. Seattle (WA): University of Washington, Seattle. Available at: https://www.ncbi.nlm.nih.gov/books/NBK1249/ [Accessed 18 November 2022].

Morris CA, Demsey SA, Leonard CO, Dilts C, Blackburn BL (1988) Natrual history of Williams syndrome: physical characteristics. *The Journal of Pediatrics* **113**: 318–326.

Murphy NA, Carbone PS (2008) Promoting the participation of children with disabilities in sports, recreation, and physical activities. *Pediatrics* **121**: 1057–1060.

Murray J, Ryan-Krause P (2010) Obesity in children with Down syndrome: background and recommendations for management. *Pediatric Nursing* **36**: 314–319. 10.1186/1472-6823-5-6.

Nordstrøm M (2015) *Obesity, Lifestyle and Cardiovascular Risk in Down Syndrome, Prader-Willi Syndrome and Williams Syndrome.* (Doctoral thesis). University of Oslo, Oslo.

O'Sullivan SB (2007) Strategies to improve motor function. In: O'Sullivan SB, Schmiz TJ, editors, *Physical Rehabilitation*, 5th ed. Philadelphia: FA Davis Company, pp 361–399.

Oppewal A, Hilgenkamp TI, van Wijck R, Evenhuis HM (2013) Cardiorespiratory fitness in individuals with intellectual disabilities: a review. *Research in Developmental Disabilities* **34**: 3301–3316.

Pless IB, Pinkerton P (1975) *Chronic Childhood Disorder: Promoting Patterns of Adjustment.* London: Kimpton.

Poirier P, Giles TD, Bray GA et al. (2006) Obesity and cardiovascular disease: pathophysiology, evaluation, and effect of weight loss an update of the 1997 American Heart Association Scientific statement on obesity and heart disease from the obesity committee of the council on nutrition, physical activity, and metabolism. *Circulation* **113**: 898–918.

Robertson J, Emerson E, Gregory N et al. (2000) Lifestyle related risk factors for poor health in residential settings for people with intellectual disabilities. *Research in Developmental Disabilites* **21**: 469–486.

Roizen N, Patterson D (2003) Down's syndrome. *The Lancet* **361**: 1281–1289.

Rosenbaum P, Gorter JW (2011) The 'F-words' in childhood disability: I swear this is how we should think! *Child: Care, Health and Development* **38**: 457–463.

Samuel A, Saxena S, Aranha V (2016) Anaerobic fitness in children with Down syndrome: a pilot cross-sectional study. *Saudi Journal of Sports Medicine* **16**: 124–127. 10.4103/1319-6308.180177.

Schalock R, Borthwick-Duffy S, Bradley V et al. (2010) *Intellectual Disability: Definition, Classification, and Systems of Support*, 11th ed. Washington: American Association on Intellectual and Developmental Disabilities.

Strømme P, Bjørnstad PG, Ramstad K (2002) Prevalence estimation of Williams syndrome. *Journal of Child Neurology* **17**: 269–271.

Thompson JR, Bradley V, Buntinx WHE et al. (2009) Conceptualizing supports and the support needs of people with intellectual disability. *Intellectual and Developmental Disabilities* **47**: 135–146.

Vogels A, Van den Ende J, Keymolen K et al. (2004) Minimum prevalence, birth incidence and mortality rate for people with Prader Willi syndrome in Flanders. *European Journal of Human Genetics* **12**: 238–240.

World Health Organization (2010) Global *Recommendations on Physical Activity for Health.* Geneva: World Health Organization.

World Health Organization (2016) Health topics [online]. Available at: http://www.euro.who.int/en/health-topics/noncommunicable-diseases/mental-health/news/news/2010/15/childrens-right-to-family-life/definition-intellectual-disability [Accessed 18 March 2022].

CHAPTER 11

Autism Spectrum Disorder

Ine Wigernaes and Ellen K Munkhaugen

This chapter begins with an overview of autism spectrum disorder (ASD), including the diagnostic criteria, prevalence, common impairments, comorbidities, and medications. This is followed by a review of the health-related fitness components of cardiorespiratory fitness and submaximal exercise capacity, muscular fitness, body composition, and flexibility. These terms are defined in Chapter 2. For each component, information on why one might wish to evaluate it, how to evaluate it, and either ASD-specific adaptation of training principles (cardiorespiratory fitness and submaximal exercise capacity, muscular fitness) or a discussion about how physical activity affects the component (body composition, flexibility) is provided. The chapter ends with an overview of guidelines on how to promote a physically active lifestyle for people with ASD exemplified with stories of lived experience.

Health-related fitness tests are classified as laboratory or field tests. Laboratory tests are often employed in research or specialized clinical contexts, while field tests are used in both research, clinical, and community settings. Chapter 2 provides a more detailed description of both these types of tests. General safety considerations are provided in Chapter 3, and general training principles and motivational factors are presented in Chapters 4 and 5.

WHAT IS ASD?

ASD is a complex heterogenous neurodevelopmental condition that is considered a lifelong disability. To have an ASD diagnosis is considered to be pervasive for the individuals, their caregivers, and their environment. Throughout this chapter, it is important to bear in mind that ASD refers to a spectrum that covers large variations in the individual's severity of symptoms, ranging from persons who are not able to speak and care for themselves to those who are able to live reasonably typical lives (Lai et al. 2014). ASD is described and referred to in the Diagnostic and Statistical Manual of Mental Disorders, Fifth Edition (American Psychiatric Association 2013) and the International Classification of Diseases, version 10 and 11 (ICD-10 and ICD-11) (see https://icd.who.int/browse10/2019/en#/). It is usually recognized in children younger than 3 years of age. Symptoms of ASD must be present in early development but may not fully manifest until social demands exceed limited capacities, such as at school age or even later in adolescence or adulthood for some persons at the more able end of the spectrum. Prominent behavioural features of ASD are impaired communication and reciprocity in social and emotional settings. There may be limitation in understanding relationships, including the intention, the values of mutual actions, and in defining their own role. The important social characteristic of non-verbal communication is usually difficult for individuals with ASD to comprehend. Restricted interests and repetitive behaviours are other core symptoms of ASD. These may include issues such as fixed interest for specific historical events or details encountered in an everyday settings. In addition, delayed motor development can sometimes be a reason for suspecting ASD (Lai et al. 2014). Motor skills range from minimal possibilities for voluntary movements to small impacts on coordination and balance. Nevertheless, gait, balance, and coordination are often affected and visibly compromised. The qualitative dysfunction within social interaction and communication, impaired ability to sense the atmosphere, context, and non-verbal communication, as well as limited stereotypical behaviour, often inhibit equal participation in play, education, and work.

Establishing an ASD diagnosis and detecting other health issues is a comprehensive process, performed by multidisciplinary teams, using a developmental framework, interviews, adaptive and cognitive assessments, and medical examination. The diagnosis is determined by summarizing observed behavioural traits within social interaction, verbal and non-verbal communication, repetitive behaviour, and restricted interests according to the criteria of the diagnostic manuals.

Weak central coherence (WCC), theory of mind, and executive functions are three theories that hypothesize ASD as a cognitive deficit (Hill 2004; Rajendran and Mitchell 2007; Happé 2022). The theories have not been able to explain unique factors that capture the heterogeneity of ASD. However, contributions from cognitive psychology have advanced our understanding, and will most probably continue to do so, in collaboration with the other disciplines involved in ASD research (Rajendran and Mitchell 2007). The WCC theory engages with the extensive focus on details that often impedes the comprehension of the total situation in persons with ASD. Separating important and non-important information may be difficult for this population (Rajendran and Mitchell 2007). This appears like a lack of natural attention directed towards obvious points of interest for others. Thus, service providers may need to help the individual to pay attention to points of interest in the present exercise or physical activity.

Theory of mind focuses on the ability to understand other's mindset or intentions (Frith and Happé 1994; Livingston et al. 2019). This 'mindlessness' impacts the understanding of social reciprocity and service providers often have to explain social rules more explicitly for the individual than for others, for example with social stories (Karkhaneh et al. 2010). Executive functions comprise several neurocognitive components including inhibition, working memory, flexibility, emotional control, initiation, planning, organization, and self-control. These components enable the individual to disengage from the present context to accomplish future goals (Hill 2004). Adherence to routines and rules often leads to resistance of changes and refusal to engage in new activities. These problems within mental flexibility are part of executive functions often present in individuals with ASD (Pellicano 2012). Deficits in all these three theories may be interpreted as lack of motivation or reluctance both to participate in the physical activity and to be with others. Thus, service providers need to be aware of these deficits and, with the individuals and their caregivers, find out how to approach new activities. Furthermore, interests and preferences need to be assessed in order to build a fitness or exercise programme around those interests while avoiding challenging issues for the individuals.

A variety of structural changes in the brain may lead to dysfunctional development. ASD is defined by a complex interaction between genetic and non-genetic factors (Lai et al. 2014). ASD has heritability at about 80% (Lai et al. 2014), but the direct cause-and-effect from specific genetic variants has yet to be elucidated. More than 1000 genes could be involved (Lai et al. 2014).

The prevalence of ASD is steadily increasing and 1 in 100 children and adolescents has ASD reported by the World Health Organization (2022), males are more often diagnosed with a 4:1 ratio (Elsabbagh et al. 2012; Xu et al. 2018; Zeidan et al. 2022). Although the severity of functional level of individuals with ASD varies largely, the need for public and personal assistance is often extensive. Even individuals who have less severe autism as children may need assistance when growing into adulthood (Howlin et al. 2013). Parents are regarded as vital to promote and encourage their children with ASD to engage in physical activity. However, this task may be too overwhelming for the parents to handle by themselves over several years. Thus, collaboration between different actors should provide assistance for the individuals with ASD (Arnell et al. 2020).

Overall, although ASD is a chronic condition, and the severity is mostly stable over the life course, early recognition, diagnosis, and treatment can improve the prognosis. Better adaptive functioning is achievable in most individuals. It is necessary to address the core deficits in ASD promoting physical activities, and providing predictability for the individuals is stated to be especially important. Further, prompting, modelling, and structured teaching using pictures and symbols and reinforcers are recommended to promote physical activity (Todd and Reid 2006; Jachyra et al. 2021). Adolescents with ASD reported that participation was positive when the physical activity was meaningful and created a purpose, a sense of identity, and met their need for affective pleasures (Menear and Neumeier 2015).

COMMON IMPAIRMENTS AND COMORBIDITIES

Associated medical and psychiatric conditions, as well as intellectual disability, may influence functioning negatively. A broad range of comorbidities is common for more than 70% of the population. The most common are sleep disorders, epileptic seizures, attention-deficit/hyperactivity disorder, gastrointestinal dysfunctions, anxiety, and depression (Lai et al. 2014; Sala et al. 2020). These comorbidities are associated with a number of negative physiological and mental outcomes, such as irritability, lower concentration, lack of initiative, obesity, diabetes, stroke, heart failure, high blood pressure, digestive problems, lower growth hormone production, and reduction of the immune function. Awareness of the numerous comorbidities needs to be targeted early in order to adapt fitness or exercise programmes to the individual needs. Furthermore, parents and the individuals themselves could inform the service provider with information about interests, sensory sensitivities, alternative and supplementary communication etc., vital to adapt and motivate the individual to participate in physical activity and to improve their overall health and well-being (Sala et al. 2020). An altered immune state is observed in ASD. A chronic neuroinflammatory state implies a larger risk of obtaining small infections, and finally total energy loss due to chronic immune reactivity. The link between nerves and the immune system could play a major role in the pathophysiology of ASD. This path needs to be further investigated (Onore et al. 2012).

In general, physical activity is known to be beneficial for the immune system. However, if physical activity becomes no longer sustainable, it may affect the immune system negatively. When the immune system is challenged by, for example, worrying, depression, inflammation, or cancer, increased attention is required when applying further stress factors, such as physical activity, travelling, temperature changes etc. Being more aware of sleeping and eating patterns and avoiding hypothermia is specifically important for a population that already faces immunological challenges (Nieman 2003).

The mortality risk is 3 to 10 times higher at any age in persons with ASD compared to a typically developed population. Causes are linked to psychical conditions as well as immune, respiratory, and gastrointestinal conditions (Sala et al. 2020).

COMMON MEDICATIONS

To date, no medications are known to improve ASD as such, or positively impact communication or social deficits. However, several drugs serve to minimize comorbidity, such as repetitive and challenging behaviour, poor sleep, intestinal problems, and epileptic seizures (Farmer et al. 2013; Lai et al. 2014).

The UK National Institute for Health and Care Excellence (NICE) guidelines are generally restrictive regarding drugs. They state that antidepressants, antipsychotics, anticonvulsants, exclusion diets (casein and gluten-free diets), or complementary supplements are not recommended for the management of core features of autism in children and young people (NICE 2017).

HOW TO ADAPT ASSESSMENTS AND INTERVENTIONS

As for diagnosing ASD, long-term interventions should be multidisciplinary and multi dimensional, in order to improve quality of life, social skills, communication, maximal functional capacity, and community engagement, and minimize maladaptive behaviours, comorbidities, and finally provide family and caregiver support. Due to the heterogeneity of ASD, an analysis of symptom severity and individual preferences and interests should therefore be the basis for treatment and services (Lai et al. 2014). Cognitive and behavioural therapy should be considered, either in groups or individually, depending on features of the condition on an individual basis (Lai et al. 2014). There is no cure for ASD. However, core symptoms may improve and comorbidities may be relieved, blunted, and even treated. Paediatricians, psychotherapists, physical and occupational therapists, and educational/clinical psychologists may all be involved (Welton, 2014; NICE 2017). Even if the pathology has a root in biology, most interventions are behavioural and educational. Physicians play an important role in coordinating care through an interdisciplinary team, referring families for specialized services and treating children's associated conditions. These include sleep disturbances, gastrointestinal problems, anxiety, overweight, and hyperactivity.

EVALUATING HEALTH-RELATED FITNESS COMPONENTS FOR PEOPLE WITH ASD

The evaluations of the components of health-related fitness as described in Chapter 4 generally require the cooperation of the individual. However, the most meaningful values will not necessarily be reference values but comparisons within the person over time. Given the enormous variation in functioning and cognition within the ASD population, specific adaptations to the tests described in Chapter 4 are not possible. Moreover, tests that require a common understanding of a timed effort and communication regarding degree of exertion will be very difficult as these factors are often severely challenged for this population. This means a correct estimate of current status of a given physical fitness component may be masked due to incomplete communication and understanding of the situation and the purpose of the test.

A pragmatic approach must therefore be taken. For cardiorespiratory endurance, it may be more feasible to measure heart rate while exercising at a certain intensity level (speed on a treadmill or speed on an exercise bicycle) and look at changes over time to get an indication of this fitness component (meaning at least over the short term, a lower heart rate at the same intensity would indicate an improvement in cardiorespiratory fitness). For muscle fitness, the functional or field tests in Chapter 4 may be more feasible and ultimately more accurate than the tests that measure these components more directly. Estimating body composition using height and weight (body mass index) and measuring flexibility with a goniometer require less voluntary activity from the individual and thus should be feasible if the person is generally cooperative and if the test is introduced slowly and perhaps practised a few times.

PROMOTING A PHYSICALLY ACTIVE LIFESTYLE IN ASD

Regular physical activity is generally described as a health-promoting factor for overall quality of life. Sedentary behaviour and low levels of physical activity are associated with short- and long-term health disadvantages in the cardiovascular, metabolic, and musculoskeletal systems. Additionally, psychosocial well-being and cognitive functioning will benefit from regular exercise compared to an inactive lifestyle. Inactivity is a strong predictor of obesity, which in turn predisposes all of us to a myriad of pathophysiological conditions. Obesity itself leads to decreased motivation for physical activity (Thomas et al. 2017). A scientific and practical approach and guideline summary towards physical activity as a beneficial intervention for children with ASD have not received much attention.

Several attempts to use exercise programmes as interventions for a variety of persons with developmental and psychiatric disorders have been reported with positive outcomes (Petrus et al. 2008). Engaging in physical activity for children with ASD may offer an arena for learning, that is, socialization with peers, minimizing obesity, and broadening interests and self-efficacy, in addition to the well-known health outcomes.

As well as traditional treatment, physical activity may be an appropriate non-pharmacological intervention. Possible improvements may include sleep patterns, repetitive behaviour, academic responses, social motivation, reciprocity, concentration, and cognition (Maglione et al. 2012; Dillon et al. 2016).

Benefits of a Physically Active Lifestyle in ASD

Most reviews on this topic request more precise methods, as the designs are weak with a low level of evidence (Dillon et al. 2016; Zarafshan et al. 2017), and there is an important research-practice gap. However, three new systematic reviews, two with meta-analyses, showed moderate to large effects of physical activity on manipulative skills, locomotor skills, skill-related fitness, social functioning, and muscular strength and endurance in young people with ASD (Healy et al. 2018). Significant positive impact was also found on social interaction ability, communication ability, and motor skills of children with ASD as well as on social and communication skills of adolescents with ASD, but no effect was shown on stereotyped behaviour (Huang et al. 2020). Results from a third systematic review supported that activity, participation, and body functions improved after physical activity interventions, and that visual instruction was more beneficial than verbal instruction (Ruggeri et al. 2020).

Nevertheless, current knowledge states that team sports may involve additional challenging situations for persons with ASD. In cognitive theory of ASD these impairments in understanding both their own and others minds are described as the theory of mind hypothesis. In team sports these impairments may impact the understanding of cooperation when playing games.

Individual activities seem to be more suitable for this group. Individual sports have shown improvements in numerous outcomes such as repetitive behaviour (Dillon et al. 2016) and social-emotional functioning, sleep, and severity of comorbidities. Horseback riding and martial arts are promising. The former has also led to less inattention and sedentary behaviour and creation of social motivation. Exercising alone was also most efficient, in terms of intensity (Dillon et al. 2016).

Exercise was reported to reduce stereotypic behaviour, and high intensity exercise shows better results than medium-/low-intensity exercise (Petrus et al. 2008). Even though the effect of high-intensity physical activity upon stereotypic behaviour is significant, the benefits are temporary in reducing inappropriate behaviour and increasing academic achievements (Petrus et al. 2008). This adds to the general list of numerous positive outcomes of physical activity interventions as 'deli-goods', that have a short life span, although still constituting important advantages. Running regularly was found to increase the perceptual and objective motor skills and also led to appropriate play, improved academic responses, and less self-stimulatory behaviour. However, speed did not improve (Rafie et al. 2017).

Other physical activities reporting positive outcomes are table tennis, which improves motor skills and executive functioning (Dillon et al. 2016); water exercise, such as swimming programmes was shown to increase aquatic skills and social behaviour (Dillon et al. 2016). Motor skills improved, as well as balance and throwing balls, after implementation of balance/coordination training and aerobic biking training. Mood and sleep objectively improved (Dillon et al. 2016). High-intensity physical activity in the morning and afternoon was reported to advance sleep phases, which may include a benefit for reducing several comorbidity challenges (Dillon et al. 2016).

Among adults with ASD, a study from USA showed that they reported more barriers and less frequent strenuous or moderate physical activity, less positive attitudes, and less perceived ease of performing physical activity compared with a comparison group. As physical activity may attenuate ASD challenges, such as anxiety, stress, and sleeping difficulties, there is a need for more physical activity for adults with ASD (Hiller et al. 2020).

Most research on physical activity in persons with ASD is conducted within individual physical activities. However, it is important to bear in mind the heterogeneity within the ASD population. As for all interventions, a systematic analysis and assessments of the individuals' needs, strengths, and preferences as well as mapping the resources in the family and the local community have to be performed. The results from such assessment might show that team sports like football and volleyball is the most preferred physical activity.

Specific Challenges in ASD

It is well known that obesity is an epidemic in Western societies, and interventions are repeatedly failing. Obesity in children, in general, is a major health concern. An overeating habit acquired as a child is likely to continue into adulthood and also descend to offspring. High body fat percentage is known to increase the risk for a number of diseases, such as diabetes, certain cancer types, cardiovascular diseases, and depression. Overweight is also a barrier for physical activity. Having a healthy and 'normal' attitude towards food and meals is important for participation in a family and a community.

Family stress, maternal depression, family cohesion, conflicts, emotional distress, and negative family interaction all influence obesity in children (Abbeduto et al. 2004; Curtin et al. 2014; Brown et al. 2020). Furthermore, the structure and energy in the family is especially crucial for lifestyle choices. Patterns of TV watching, games, food selection, meal behaviour, and family cooking together are known variables, and parent support in establishment of routines including physical activity should be emphasized (Brown et al. 2020).

In the USA, overweight is defined as having a sex-specific body mass index for age greater than the 85th centile. Obesity relates to the population that has a body mass index for age at or above the 95th centile (Abbeduto et al. 2004; Curtin et al. 2014).

People with ASD also have a higher risk for being obese than their age-matched peers. In a recent review, 20% to 25% of males with ASD were obese. In females, the number was significantly lower (Curtin et al. 2014). A definitive genetic association between ASD and obesity is not known. However, genetic duplications and deletions at gene 16p11.2 are commonly connected to ASD. This sequence has also been shown to play a role in childhood obesity (Abbeduto et al. 2004; Curtin et al. 2014).

Children with ASD have a higher degree of food selectivity (picky eaters) than typically developing children. These children eat less fruit and vegetables compared to typically developing peers (Abbeduto et al. 2004; Curtin et al. 2014). The link between high-level intake of sugar sweetened beverages and a lower intake of fruit and vegetables in relation to obesity is also well known, and may also apply for this population. In families with children with an ASD diagnosis, mealtimes may be especially important as a social venue where social values such as reciprocal behaviour, communication skills, and appropriate behaviour may be learned (Abbeduto et al. 2004; Curtin et al. 2014).

There is a high prevalence of sleep problems in children with ASD (Abbeduto et al. 2004; Curtin et al. 2014). There is an established link between short duration of sleep and increased body weight and obesity (Abbeduto et al. 2004; Curtin et al. 2014). Decreased leptin levels are a well-known result of poor sleep and induce an increase in appetite (Abbeduto et al. 2004; Curtin et al. 2014). Energy balance throughout the day is often severely affected and can lead to lower motivation for engaging in activities. For children with ASD, there is little data on sleep. Intuitively, the established knowledge of compromised sleep pattern for children with ASD is likely also to cause decreased leptin levels also in this population.

The majority of typically developing children do not meet the criteria for daily physical activity. It is agreed that children with ASD are less physically active than peers and thus even fewer meet national recommendation/guidelines (Abbeduto et al. 2004; Curtin et al. 2014). This population spends less time in vigorous activity while playing free play and also does fewer activities compared to typically developing children (Abbeduto et al. 2004; Curtin et al. 2014). ASD and intellectual impairment expose people with disabilities at a higher risk for sedentariness. It has been shown that the association between physical activity and quality of life is underestimated in children with ASD and their families (Abbeduto et al. 2004; Curtin et al. 2014).

Numerous and more complex additional barriers exist for children with ASD. The inherent impaired social and communication skills and the rigid and stereotypical behaviour were mentioned earlier. Additionally, factors like time constraints, transportation, communication, access, limited motor skills, inappropriate behaviour, and motivation are identified by parents (Must et al. 2015). Parents' engagement in physical activity may actually predict children's participation.

Not surprisingly, negative experiences are antecedents for sedentary behaviour (Dillon et al. 2016). Poor motor skills are demotivating for all people, including for those diagnosed with ASD. Unevenness in developmental milestone acquisition, low muscle tone, and poor balance constitute true barriers for motivation, mastering experiences, or creating self-efficacy (Dillon et al. 2016).

There is also a known positive connection between cheerfulness, satisfaction, and participation for this group. Lack of positive experiences, frequent failures, emotional impairments, low self-esteem, and low self-efficacy contribute to a negative spiral. In combination with low income, the barrier becomes even larger.

Lower cardiac responses to different tests for children with ASD, as compared to typically developing children, have been shown (Pace and Bricout 2015). No scientific materials discuss the issue of how children with ASD understand a command of 'maximum effort', as in a handgrip or jump maximal test procedure.

Parent reports or accelerometers are usually used to measure levels of activity. Measuring screen time is interesting as opposed to measuring exercise time exclusively. In a recent study, two groups were compared: 53 children with ASD and 58 typically developing children participated. Lack of adult skills, few friends, characteristics of the disability, and exclusion of their child were the most highlighted barriers reported from parents of autistic children. Parent-reported barriers were significantly inversely related to hours of physical activity and positively related to screen time (Must et al. 2015). More screen time and less activity time have been observed. Males are more active than females, which may be explained by there being more females with severe ASD.

It is important to be reminded about the enormous variation of severity of symptoms; however, motor skills and balance difficulties are some of the common features in autistic children. This is a true challenge for these young people when engaging in physical activity. Stereotypic motion disturbances, lack of social skills, and difficulties in understanding social interplay may also be factors for a higher threshold and lower motivation for initiating and continuing participation.

CONCLUSIONS

Human, organizational, and facility resources required to implement successful non-pharmacological interventions are high. Nevertheless, physical activity interventions have explicit benefits in terms of their non-pharmacological, non-invasive nature and lack of side-effects.

There are numerous positive outcomes of physical activity for individuals with ASD, but evidence is currently limited. Physical activity in one form or another is beneficial, as opposed to inactivity. Health professionals and cross-sectional teams need to acknowledge that the social and health-related benefits should be a target for people with ASD as well as others. Similar to behavioural and educational interventions applied, caregivers should also be involved. Children's preferences for the type of physical activity also need to be taken into account. Setting realistic goals that are measurable for those involved is of great importance. Involving significant and dedicated others is important for caregivers. Lifestyle intervention has explicit benefits in terms of its non-pharmacological, non-invasive nature and lack of side-effects.

The energy and effort spent by parents in handling their child's ASD may prevent them from dedicating time to physical activity. The child's limitation may be another cause. Access and lack of suitable facilities are reported as major barriers. The multidisciplinary teams may strive to incorporate social and participating goals beyond lean body mass, targeting heart rate and healthier blood pressure. It seems that improving motivation by targeting and encouraging parents' engagement in physical activity in the interventions may lead to even more participation, and will lead to more interesting research results for this large population.

Similar to the general population, persons with ASD add to the trend that few people meet the recommendation of daily physical activity. It is a goal to break the cycle of inactivity. In this chapter, we have described some of the 'keys'. Searching for motivation for long-term adherence and change is one of the most important factors. What motivates individuals varies through age and situations, physical and mental conditions. This requires a highly individual approach. A structural and critical identification of barriers and the individual's wishes must be performed. A change always requires extra energy. Sticking to the plan and the daily or weekly habit is crucial. Improving the individual's physical well-being should be prioritized.

STORIES OF LIVED EXPERIENCE

The Caregivers' Search for Facilities

A highly educated mother is at a rehabilitation centre with her 14-year-old son, Martin, at a 3-week stay for the third time. The main intervention at this centre is adapted physical activity and socialization in groups with children/young people with a wide range of disabilities. Martin is the only one in the group of 10 with ASD. With some assistance, he attends a secondary school for typically developing children.

Everyday Behaviour

Martin's mother underlines her emphasis of teaching him how his behaviour may be offending, strange, or scary to others. 'I can teach him everything as long as I manage to exemplify and relate to his own experience as soon as possible. I can tell him that I saw someone being sorry after something he said. Then I tell him to take a different approach next time, and his friend will not be this sorry.'

Everyday tasks, like dining together and seeing friends, are opportunies for all kinds of development. She explains: 'I can tell him that "Good job, Martin, you were really good with the baby today. Did you see how happy the mum and the baby were when you helped the baby out with the toy?"' Martin learns about social interplay, but she is sure her son will never fully understand the concept. 'But it is a blessing that I am able to teach him, train him, on a repetitive manner, the volume of speech, face expressions, and polite behaviour. And it works. He does not want to hurt anyone, and the development into wanting to use an appropriate language is growing by age.' When she has taught him to wait for her somewhere, he will be there no matter how much time it takes. She also experiences that he will never forget the mission, and he acts like he is taught and shows that he is learning.

In the Rehabilitation Setting

The mother is crystal clear about the effect of being with other kids with different chronic challenges. 'The atmosphere is tolerant and generous,' she says.

This applies also to the health professionals. Introducing new group activities in an unfamiliar environment with unknown peers is a major issue for children with autism. 'At his local school, for typically developing children, he attends and accepts following his peers on physical and cultural activities but never performs or enjoys or repeats them. His slow articulation and speech are a challenge. At his home community, the only one listening to him is a friend in a wheelchair, who has the patience. The other classmates are gone before he has finished the first sentence in his story.'

While his peers play football, he cannot understand the game, the purpose, the meaning, or his role. Here at the rehabilitation centre, he is given more time and is listened to. Then he relaxes. 'I attribute this completely to the attitude and setting of this rehabilitation centre,' his mother says. The health professionals just lead him gently into activities, without any demands.

'I wonder why I am here,' he says. 'Most of the others are in a wheelchair, how come I am allowed to be here?' His mother has never told her son that he has autism. Nevertheless, he is aware of being different from the rest. This is the fourth time they have attended this specific rehabilitation programme. Even the first time, the new routines did not include all the challenges that she anticipated. I think the culture of welcoming different people with different challenges was so obvious that even a 10-year-old boy with autism was able to accept dining rooms, group activities, and new people.

The Athlete With Autism

Martin's mother credits the rehabilitation stay for creating lots of energy and construction of mastering experiences and self-efficacy during the first rehabilitation stay. Prior to this, Martin was never engaged in any sport activities. The motivation was not there. 'After the first rehabilitation stay he wanted to push himself. The extra energy needed a channel, and I knew I had to move quickly,' his mother remembers.

A friend introduced her to the idea of rowing competition activities. 'While entering the local rowing club we were calmed down when being approached by the same generous attitude,' she explains. There were never more than 25 rowers attending the exercise sessions. 'My son is in a total flow. The tasks in a rowing competition are simple. When in front, he is the one to initiate the first 10 strokes. When passing the 500m mark, he has learned to initiate another rhythm, and finally, he gives a new command for the last 250m before crossing the line.' Rowing is rhythmical and there are three tasks along the competition. Martin is fortunate as he is never affected by the seriousness of the competition, foreign countries, expectations, or the media. 'He sticks to the plan and performs the exercises he has learned again and again,' his mother smiles.

This strategy and this approach is exactly what typically developing athletes strive to achieve with their mindset when competitions are coming up. Suddenly, autism becomes an advantage. 'We need to keep searching intensively for opportunities for each person with ASD in order to improve quality of life and create good situations. Of course, this is a breakthrough and lifts the total energy in the family, and my life,' she smiles.

A 3-WEEK REHABILITATION PROGRAMME EMPHASIZING ADAPTED PHYSICAL ACTIVITY: CHALLENGES, EXPERIENCES, AND DILEMMAS

With 50 years of experience in using physical activity as a main tool in rehabilitation of a population of adults with chronic physical disabilities, Beitostølen Health Sport Center in Norway started to offer rehabilitation for children and young people with ASD in 2010.

A group approach, an unfamiliar place, remotely situated in the foothills of the national park of the highest mountains in the country, with more than 100 employees, 70 patients, open areas, physical activity in three to five bouts per day in new exercises, new equipment, and new facilities may not seem to be either suitable or desired for this population. There is consensus, based on the main features of this disability, that there is a need for a high level of predictability, familiar places, and personnel (Lai et al. 2014). In addition, impaired motor control, aggression, and the lack of socialization, reciprocity, and communication skills could oppose or at least hinder the team-work process, and are other reasons for not encouraging such a rehabilitation programme.

However, summarizing the experiences, the most appropriate description within this group of patients is the extent of variation. Many years of experience have taught the professionals that with adaptation efforts and extra focus, one person with ASD in a rehabilitation group of 10 children usually works fine. Adding another person with similar challenges usually works poorly. The group focus for the remaining children and young people with several disabilities would be severely compromised, in terms of behavioural problems, noise, and aggression. This requires the occupation of health personnel in a one-to-one capacity, instead of participation in activities together, in a group, which serves as a base for this rehabilitation approach.

When children and young people with ASD meet others with the same diagnosis, it is usually fruitful. Watching how the older ones can manage social skills and communication is an unambiguous positive experience, especially for caregivers. Returning for rehabilitation programmes the second and third time constitutes, without exception, an improvement from the first time, underlining the value of experience, expectation, familiarity, the feeling of security, and predictability.

The programme personnel usually try to inform the family of the plans prior to the activities. This includes a thorough introduction of the complete setting, and description of halls, training facilities, and equipment. They also seek to reduce the number of personnel per individual with ASD to two. Changes will nevertheless be a part of the rehabilitation programme. No matter how specifically the teams try to prepare the group and their caregivers, unexpected events occur. Another message from experienced professionals is that information that is too detailed may be perceived as changes and unexpected events. Therefore, balanced information is important.

The personnel discuss their efforts to accommodate the desire for predictability as opposed to preparing the young persons with ASD for a life outside rehabilitation. This presents a dilemma between the wish for plans and predictability versus preparing the children and young people for participating in education, work, social events, and independent living. This point should be thoroughly discussed in practice settings when initiating programmes for a population with ASD – namely, the purpose within the rehabilitation context versus what happens in the real world. These two positive intentions may not always overlap in ways that are mutually beneficial.

Illustrating Stories

An excavator or a large truck totally occupied a 10-year-old boy for 2 weeks. The rehabilitation process was never initiated.

A girl who re-entered the Healthsports centre for rehabilitation after 2 years really looked forward to meeting the horse Daisy again. Meanwhile, the old horse Daisy had passed away. This fact kept her distressed for more than 1 week into rehabilitation.

The boy loved the bike he tried out and rode all Wednesday. On Thursday, the bike was occupied when he came to borrow it. This occurrence swept him off his feet. Trying another more expensive, newer bike was out of the question.

Cross-country skiing was a great experience for a boy, until he was passed by a random skier. The event led to a total breakdown and massive efforts were needed to retry the next day.

One physical education instructor had established circuit training in a gym for strengthening upper and lower body, abdominals, hip, and shoulder/back for several children with ASD. After 9 weeks doing the same exercises, an instinct for most people is being afraid of the repetition becoming boring. Accordingly, and with positive intentions, she introduced new exercises. The change was not well-received. There was a point where she wondered if her positive intention had the potential to ruin the whole concept of circuit training and exceptional trust in the group that she had built during the spring. She rebuilt the circuit system into the old exercises. Slowly, the group got back on track, with better mood and with high motivation and pleasure.

A 14-year-old boy had barely learned to swim. To make him more competent, the personnel tried to teach him how to improve strokes for security and comfort in the water. He denied and ignored all kinds of hints aggressively. The efforts were automatically transformed into an unambiguous negative critique. The bottom line is that small defeats may have proportionally larger negative consequences for children with ASD than for children and young people with other kinds of disabilities.

The head of the horse instructors met a 9-year-old girl in the preparing and dressing room at the stable. She was constantly looking down, even while approaching her personally. A short standard introduction was performed. It turned out that for this girl, trying on a helmet was unthinkable. Looking into the stable with the horses was totally out of the question. The instructor improvised. She owned a dog and rapidly fetched it and asked if the girl wanted to take the dog out for a walk on a leash. For the first time the girl looked her shyly in the eyes and replied almost inaudibly, 'yes'. After 20 minutes, the girl returned as a totally different person, smiling, laughing, talking constantly about the details of the experience; the dog's behaviour, the petting and hugging, and meeting people and insects. She held the instructor's gaze for a long time, and articulated loud and clear. Not long after, she enjoyed approaching a horse.

The 10-year-old boy spent the entire week watching the other children on the playground trying out different kinds of cycling equipment depending on their disability. The professionals were unsure what to do. They weighed encouragement against pushing, impatience to teach versus knowledge that kids with ASD need more time. In his way, he participated and communicated, but he showed no sign of wanting to try riding a bicycle in the 7 days. On the eighth day, he firmly walked to the bicycle storage room, selected a bike, and started cycling, with perfect technique, turns, and a great smile.

In summary, both research and current practice show that physical activity interventions are beneficial and necessary for people with ASD, as for everybody else. Continuous physical activity seems to be most beneficial both for health, activity skills, and participation ability.

REFERENCES

Abbeduto L, Seltzer MM, Shattuck P, Krauss MW, Orsmond G, Murphy MM (2004) Psychological well-being and coping in mothers of youths with autism, Down syndrome, or fragile X syndrome. *Am J Ment Retard* **109**: 237–254.

Thomas DT, Erdman KA, Burke LM (2017) American College of Sports Medicine joint position statement: nutrition and athletic performance. *Med Sci Sports Exerc* **48**: 543–568.

American Psychiatric Association (2013) *Diagnostic and Statistical Manual of Mental Disorders, Fifth Edition*. Arlington, VA: American Psychiatric Association.

Arnell S, Jerlinder K, Lundqvist L-O (2020) Parents' perceptions and concerns about physical activity participation among adolescents with autism spectrum disorder. *Autism* 24: 2243–2255.

Brand S, Jossen S, Holsboer-Trachsler E, Puhse U, Gerber M (2015) Impact of aerobic exercise on sleep and motor skills in children with autism spectrum disorders: a pilot study. *Neuropsychiatr Dis Treat* 11: 1911–1920.

Brown DM, Arbour-Nicitopoulos KP, Martin Ginis KA, Latimer-Cheung AE, Bassett-Gunter RL (2020) Examining the relationship between parent physical activity support behaviour and physical activity among children and youth with autism spectrum disorder. *Autism* 24: 1783–1794.

Curtin C, Jojic M, Bandini LG (2014) Obesity in children with autism spectrum disorder. *Harv Rev Psychiatry* 22: 93–103.

Dillon SR, Adams D, Goudy L, Bittner M, McNamara S (2016) Evaluating exercise as evidence-based practice for individuals with autism spectrum disorder. *Front Public Health* 4: 290.

Elsabbagh M, Divan G, Koh YJ et al. (2012) Global prevalence of autism and other pervasive developmental disorders. *Autism Res* 5: 160–179.

Farmer C, Thurm A, Grant P (2013) Pharmacotherapy for the core symptoms in autistic disorder: current status of the research. *Drugs* 73: 303–314.

Frith U, Happé F (1994) Autism: beyond 'theory of mind'. Cognition 50: 115–132.

Happé F (2022) Weak central coherence in adults with ASD: Evidence from eye-tracking and thematic content analysis of social scenes. *Appl Neuropsychol Adult* 2022: 1–12.

Healy S, Nacario A, Braitwaite RE, Hopper C (2018) The effect of physical activity interventions on youth with autism spectrum disorder: a meta-analysis. *Autism Research* 11: 818–833.

Hill EL (2004) Executive dysfunction in autism. *Trends Cogn Sci* 8: 26–32.

Hiller A, Buckingham A, Schena D (2020) Physical activity among adults with autism: participation, attitudes, and barriers. *Perceptual and Motor Skills* 127: 874–890.

Howlin P, Moss P, Savage S, Rutter M (2013) Social outcomes in mid- to later adulthood among individuals diagnosed with autism and average nonverbal IQ as children. *J Am Acad Child Adolesc Psychiatry* 52: 572–81.e1.

Huang J, Chunjie Du C, Liu J, Tan G (2020) Review meta-analysis on intervention effects of physical activities on children and adolescents with autism. *Int J Environ Res Public Health* 17: 1950.

Jachyra P, Renwick R, Gladstone B, Anagnostou E, Gibson BE (2021) Physical activity participation among adolescents with autism spectrum disorder. *Autism* 25: 613–626.

Karkhaneh M, Clark B, Ospina MB, Seida JC, Smith V, Hartling L (2010) Social Stories™ to improve social skills in children with autism spectrum disorder: a systematic review. *Autism* 14: 641–662.

Lai MC, Lombardo MV, Baron-Cohen S (2014) Autism. *Lancet* 383: 896–910.

Livingston LA, Colvert E, Team SRS, Bolton P, Happé F (2019) Good social skills despite poor theory of mind: exploring compensation in autism spectrum disorder. *Journal of Child Psychology and Psychiatry* 60: 102–110.

Maglione MA, Gans D, Das L, Timbie J, Kasari C (2012) Nonmedical interventions for children with ASD: recommended guidelines and further research needs. *Pediatrics* 130: S169–178.

Menear KS, Neumeier WH (2015) Promoting physical activity for students with autism spectrum disorder: barriers, benefits, and strategies for success. *Journal of Physical Education, Recreation and Dance* **86**: 43–48.

Must A, Phillips S, Curtin C, Bandini LG (2015) Barriers to physical activity in children with autism spectrum disorders: relationship to physical activity and screen time. *J Phys Act Health* **12**: 529–534.

NICE (2017) *Autism Spectrum Disorder in Adults: Diagnosis and Management* [online]. Available at: https://pathways.nice.org.uk/pathways/autism-spectrum-disorder [Accessed 2017].

Nieman DC (2003) Current perspective on exercise immunology. *Curr Sports Med Rep* **2**: 239–242.

Onore C, Careaga M, Ashwood P (2012) The role of immune dysfunction in the pathophysiology of autism. *Brain Behav Immun* **26**: 383-392.

Pace M, Bricout VA (2015) Low heart rate response of children with autism spectrum disorders in comparison to controls during physical exercise. *Physiol Behav* **141**: 63–68.

Pellicano E (2012) The development of executive function in autism. *Autism Research and Treatment* **2012**: 146132.

Apetrus C, Adamson SR, Block L, Einarson SJ, Sharifnejad M, Harris SR (2008) Effects of exercise interventions on stereotypic behaviours in children with autism spectrum disorder. *Physiother Can* **60**: 134–145.

Rafie F, Ghasemi A, Zamani Jam A, Jalali S (2017) Effect of exercise intervention on the perceptual-motor skills in adolescents with autism. *J Sports Med Phys Fitness* **57**: 53–59.

Rajendran G, Mitchell P (2007) Cognitive theories of autism. *Developmental Review* **27**: 224–260.

Ruggeri A, Dancel A, Johnson R, Sargent B (2020) The effect of motor and physical activity intervention on motor outcomes of children with autism spectrum disorder: a systematic review. *Autism* **24**: 544–568.

Sala R, Amet L, Blagojevic-Stokic N, Shattock P, Whiteley PJND (2020) Bridging the gap between physical health and autism spectrum disorder. *Neuropsychiatr Dis Treat* **16**: 1605–1618.

Todd T, Reid G (2006) Increasing physical activity in individuals with autism. *Focus on Autism and other Developmental Disabilities* **21**: 167–176.

Welton J (2014) *Can I Tell You about Autism?: A Guide for Friends, Family and Professionals.* London: Jessica Kingsley Publishers.

World Health Organization (2022) *Autism* [online]. Available at: https://www.who.int/news-room/fact-sheets/detail/autism-spectrum-disorders [Accessed 17 November 2022].

Xu G, Stratnearn L, Liu B, Bao W (2018) Prevalence of autism spectrum disorder among US children and adolescents, 2014–2016. *JAMA* **319**: 81–82.

Zarafshan H, Salmanian M, Aghamohammadi S, Mohammadi MR, Mostafavi SA (2017) Effectiveness of non-pharmacological interventions on stereotyped and repetitive behaviors of preschool children with autism: a systematic review. *Basic Clin Neurosci* **8**: 95–103.

Zeidan J, Fombonne E, Scorah J et al. (2022) Global prevalence of autism: a systematic review update. *Autism Res* **15**: 778–790.

CHAPTER 12

Juvenile Idiopathic Arthritis

Kristine Risum

This chapter begins with a description of juvenile idiopathic arthritis (JIA), including common medications, impairments, and comorbidities. This is followed by a presentation of the components of health-related fitness, cardiorespiratory fitness and submaximal exercise capacity, muscular fitness, body composition, and flexibility. Definitions of these terms are found in Chapter 2. The reasons why and how to evaluate these components are noted for each of them. Finally, specific training principles for people with JIA (cardiorespiratory fitness and submaximal exercise capacity, muscular fitness) and how physical activity affects the components, body composition, and particularly flexibility are described. In conclusion, suggestions for promoting a physically active lifestyle for people with JIA are discussed, in addition to specific precautions regarding periods with high disease activity, involvement of heart and lungs, and use of long-term or high doses of systemic corticosteroids.

The tests used to evaluate each health-related fitness component are classed as laboratory or field tests. Laboratory tests are typically used in research or specialized clinical settings, whereas field tests can be used in research, clinical, and community settings. Chapter 2 includes a more detailed description of both types of tests, Chapter 3 describes general safety considerations, and Chapters 4 and 5 include general training principles and motivational factors for a physically active lifestyle.

WHAT IS JIA?

JIA is the most common paediatric rheumatic condition, and it affects approximately one in 1000 people internationally. JIA is characterized by arthritis (inflammation of the joints) of unknown cause in one or more joints that persists for more than

6 weeks and with onset before 16 years of age (Prakken et al. 2011). According to the International League of Associations for Rheumatology classification criteria of JIA there are seven categories related to the number of joints affected and the presence of additional symptoms (Petty et al. 2004) (see Table 12.1). Of the International League

Table 12.1 The International League of Associations for Rheumatology criteria for the classification of juvenile idiopathic arthritis

Systemic arthritis	Arthritis and fever for at least 2 weeks. There is often skin rash and it may cause inflammation of internal organs, including the heart, liver, spleen, and lymph nodes.
Oligoarthritis	Oligo = few.
	Arthritis affecting 1–4 joints during the first 6 months after onset of the condition.
	Two subcategories:
	Persistent oligoarthritis; affecting 1–4 joints throughout the course of the condition.
	Extended oligoarthritis; affecting more than 4 joints after the first 6 months following the onset of the condition.
Rheumatoid factor-negative polyarthritis	Poly = many.
	Arthritis affecting 5 or more joints during the first 6 months after onset of the condition and negative test for rheumatoid factor (examined by blood test).
Rheumatoid factor-positive polyarthritis	Arthritis affecting 5 or more joints during the first 6 months after onset of the condition and 2 or more tests positive for rheumatoid factor (examined by blood test) at least 3 months apart during the first 6 months after onset of the condition.
Psoriasis arthritis	Arthritis and psoriasis (skin rash), or arthritis and at least 2 of the following:
	• inflammation in finger or toe
	• pits or ridges in fingernails
	• a first-degree relative with psoriasis.
Enthesitis-related arthritis	Arthritis and enthesitis (inflammation where the tendons or ligaments attach to the bones), or arthritis or enthesitis with 2 of the following:
	• the presence of or a history of sacroiliac joint tenderness and/or inflammatory spinal pain
	• presence of human lymphocyte antigen B27
	• onset of arthritis in a male >6y of age
	• acute anterior uveitis (eye inflammation)
	• a first-degree relative with a history of ankylosing spondylitis, enthesitis-related arthritis, sacroiliitis with inflammatory bowel disease, Reiter syndrome, or acute anterior uveitis.
Undifferentiated arthritis	Arthritis that fulfils criteria in no category or in 2 or more of the above categories.

of Associations for Rheumatology JIA categories, children with persistent oligoarticular JIA (one to four affected joints) are most likely to achieve remission (no disease activity or symptoms), while children with polyarticular rheumatoid factor-positive JIA are least likely to achieve remission followed by children with enthesitis-related arthritis (in which there is inflammation at tendon-to-bone insertion sites) (Shoop-Worrall et al. 2017).

JIA is an autoimmune condition, meaning that the immune system reacts against the individual's own body; yet the causes of JIA are still poorly understood. It is hypothesized that a genetically susceptible individual could develop an uncontrolled and harmful immune response towards a self-antigen after exposure to an unknown environmental trigger (Giancane et al. 2017). The disease encompasses a wide variety of patients and the disease activity can vary from one episode with arthritis in one joint to arthritis in several joints acquiring treatment into adulthood (Prakken et al. 2011). Arthritis leads to swelling and often pain and stiffness of the affected joints. Extra-articular manifestations include enthesitis, psoriasis (skin disease), uveitis (eye inflammation), and systemic features like high spiking fever (Prakken et al. 2011). These impairments may contribute to limited physical functioning in daily life and limited participation in leisure activities and sports (Cavallo et al. 2015).

COMMON IMPAIRMENTS AND COMORBIDITIES

The most common symptoms of JIA include joint swelling, stiffness, particularly morning stiffness, and pain, and children may also experience fatigue (Prakken et al. 2011). The swelling of the joints is caused by inflammation of the synovium (tissue lining around a joint, which produces fluid helping the joints to move smoothly). In JIA, the synovial lining produces increased amounts of synovial fluid (Rigante et al. 2015). Thus, reduced range of motion in joints can occur in affected joints, which subsequently can cause muscle atrophy (loss of muscle tissue) near affected joints (Klepper et al. 2019).

Taken together, these symptoms may affect how children with JIA are able to move their bodies in everyday life. These symptoms and limitations are most often present at the onset of the condition and flares. Children who use systemic glucocorticoids in high doses for long periods are at risk of developing osteoporosis (loss of bony tissue), which is most common in children with systemic onset JIA. Vitamin D supplements are important in such cases (Prakken et al. 2011). Also, recent research has reported that JIA may be associated with suspected risk of developing future cardiovascular disease (Bohr et al. 2016).

Importantly, the multidisciplinary management of JIA has improved the outcomes of JIA dramatically, and more children achieve remission, fewer children develop severe functional limitations, and more children may participate in physical activities with their peers (Shoop-Worrall et al. 2017; Risum et al. 2018). However, having JIA may still cause impairments in cardiorespiratory fitness, muscular fitness, body composition, and flexibility, and will be discussed specifically in the following section.

COMMON MEDICATIONS

International medical treatment guidelines suggest early and aggressive medical treatment to manage inflammation and optimally achieve remission (Ringold et al. 2013, 2019). The first-line treatment for most JIA categories includes non-steroidal anti-inflammatory drugs to reduce pain and inflammation, and traditional disease-modifying anti-rheumatic drugs (DMARDs) to modify the course of the disease. Methotrexate is the most used traditional DMARD in the management of JIA. Biological DMARDs are used in moderately or more severely affected patients when other treatment is not working optimally. These agents are designed to selectively block signalling molecules involved in the inflammatory process in JIA. The introduction of biological DMARDs in the new millennium has revolutionized the treatment of JIA. Biological DMARDs are recommended for use in combination with traditional DMARDs. Additionally, glucocorticoid joint injections and occasionally systemic glucocorticoids may also be used to manage pain and inflammation (Ringold et al. 2013, 2019).

CARDIORESPIRATORY FITNESS AND SUBMAXIMAL EXERCISE CAPACITY

Most studies of children with JIA have found poor cardiorespiratory fitness in children with JIA compared to typically developing peers, both measured directly and estimated through performance on maximal and submaximal tests (Maggio et al. 2010; Van Pelt et al. 2012). Associations between cardiorespiratory fitness and disease variables have not been extensively examined, but cardiorespiratory fitness is reported to be lowest in patients with active disease. Low cardiorespiratory fitness is also present in patients in remission (Van Pelt et al. 2012). A recent study that exclusively included children with JIA who were diagnosed after the introduction of biological DMARDs found similar cardiorespiratory fitness (VO$_{2peak}$ measured directly) between children with JIA and typically developing children (Risum et al. 2019). Further, there were no associations between disease-related factors and cardiorespiratory fitness in children with JIA, but higher cardiorespiratory fitness was associated with male sex, lower body mass index (BMI), and higher levels of physical activity of vigorous intensity, all factors that are well recognized for higher cardiorespiratory fitness in typically developing children (Risum et al. 2019).

The recently reported risk for cardiovascular diseases in JIA underlines the importance of focusing on exercise and physical activities that improve cardiorespiratory fitness in these children.

How to Evaluate the Cardiorespiratory Fitness and Submaximal Exercise Capacity of People With JIA

Laboratory Tests

In laboratory or research settings, direct measurement of oxygen uptake through a maximal treadmill or bicycle test is used. Bicycle tests may provide less stress on the joints in the lower extremities compared to treadmill tests, yet many children are capable of performing a treadmill test as well. Availability of equipment will often determine the choice of test.

Field Tests

Submaximal tests do not reach the maximum of the respiratory or cardiovascular systems, and are not performed at the highest possible level of exertion. The 6-minute walk test is probably the most commonly used submaximal test in JIA. However, the 6-minute walk test is reported to be a poor predictor of cardiorespiratory fitness (VO_{2peak}), and rather a measure of walking capacity in children with JIA (Lelieveld et al. 2005).

Bicycle tests are also extensively used to measure cardiorespiratory fitness in JIA. One example is the Åstrand test, which is a submaximal bicycle test. Bicycle tests may provide less stress on the joints in the lower extremities compared to treadmill tests and walking tests on the floor, and could be considered in children with active arthritis or pain in the lower extremities. Yet many children with JIA are also able to perform walking tests and treadmill tests without difficulties. Availability of equipment and the child's preferences should be taken into account if measurement of cardiorespiratory fitness is relevant for a particular child.

In addition, cardiorespiratory fitness impairments may be screened by observing the performance of activities such as brisk walking, jumping, or climbing stairs. Such observation may be particularly relevant when it is not possible to use standardized tests such as those mentioned above. This can be the case especially with very young children with JIA.

JIA-Specific Training Principles for Cardiorespiratory Fitness

In general, the training principles for typically developing children to improve cardiorespiratory fitness (see Chapter 2) apply for children with JIA as well. Many children with JIA may participate in the same physical activities as typically developing peers to improve cardiorespiratory fitness. In case of active arthritis or joint pain, or when having experienced prolonged physically inactivity, cardiorespiratory fitness training may be easier to accomplish by bicycling, swimming, or walking and running on soft surfaces to reduce the joint loading. Importantly, playing both unorganized as well as organized physical activity (ball play/sports and dancing) may improve cardiorespiratory fitness.

MUSCULAR FITNESS (MUSCLE STRENGTH AND MUSCLE ENDURANCE)

Muscle atrophy and weakness are most pronounced in muscles surrounding joints with active arthritis but may persist after clinical resolution of inflammation (Lindehammar and Lindvall 2004). The evidence on muscular fitness and endurance in children with JIA compared to typically developing children is somewhat conflicting, but most studies have reported lower muscle strength in patients with JIA compared to controls (Saarinen et al. 2008; Risum et al. 2019). Regarding hand strength, the majority of patients with JIA have normal strength in the hands, but some patients, especially those with polyarthritis and arthritis in the hands, had reduced hand muscle strength (Lindehammar 2003). Studies have used different measurement methods to assess muscle strength, even though most studies have measured muscle strength by some kind of isometric dynamometers (se Chapter 2). Also, different muscle groups have been tested, making it difficult to compare results across studies.

Knowledge about associations between muscle strength and endurance and disease variables in children with JIA is sparse. A recent study that exclusively included children with JIA who were diagnosed after the introduction of biological DMARDs found no associations between disease-related factors and muscle strength in children with JIA, but higher muscle strength was associated with male sex, higher BMI, and higher levels of physical activity of vigorous intensity, all factors that are well recognized for higher muscle strength in typically developing children (Risum et al. 2019).

How to Evaluate the Muscular Fitness of People With JIA

LABORATORY TESTS

To measure muscle fitness in children with JIA in laboratory or research settings, a handheld dynamometer or handgrip dynamometer are mostly used. Isokinetic testing for the assessment of both muscle strength and endurance has been less used, but has been applied in some research studies. See Chapter 2 for more information about the measurement methods.

FIELD TESTS

To measure muscle fitness in children with JIA with field tests or in clinical care, several tests are available. Both manual muscle testing and handgrip dynamometer are widely used. Further, observation of the child's muscle strength and endurance may be evaluated by the performance of different activities (e.g. walking, squatting, jumping, and climbing), which may be particularly relevant in preschoolers and younger children. In older children with JIA, the number of repetitions performed on different tests may be useful (e.g. push-ups and sit-ups).

JIA-Specific Training Principles for Muscular Fitness

In general, the training principles for typically developing children to improve muscular fitness (see Chapter 2) apply for children with JIA as well. Many children with JIA may participate in the same physical activities as typically developing peers to improve muscular fitness. In the case of active arthritis or joint pain, or when having had prolonged physically inactivity, some precautions should be considered. Initially, it is recommended to start with a low to moderate load and many repetitions and gradually increase the load and reduce the number of repetitions. Attention to possible increased joint swelling or joint pain is important, and adaptation may be necessary if such symptoms occur after training. However, it is normal to experience delayed muscle soreness after initiating muscle fitness training in untrained individuals, in both children with JIA and typically developing peers.

In preschoolers and young schoolchildren with JIA, training of muscle strength and endurance might best be performed by participating in physical activities that strengthens the muscles during natural play and other activities of the child's daily life rather than prescribed exercise therapy programmes.

Older children and adolescents with JIA may perform strength training by using body weight exercises, machines, or free weights. Such strength training in persons with JIA should initially be guided by experienced and educated health care or fitness professionals to ensure appropriate training technique to avoid injuries or overloading of the joints.

BODY COMPOSITION (INCLUDING BONE MINERAL DENSITY)

There is scarce knowledge of body composition in JIA and the results are conflicting. In children with JIA both comparable, lower and higher fat mass, and lower and normal lean mass compared to typically developing controls have been reported (Houttu et al. 2020). Fat mass (tissue) produces proinflammatory signalling molecules (Li et al. 2017) that may negatively influence the disease activity in JIA. Thus, emphasis on normal body composition is particularly important in JIA, and having a physically active lifestyle may be an important contribution regarding this goal.

Bone mineral density (the amount of bone mineral in bones) is an important component of body composition in JIA. Most studies find there is lower bone mineral density in children with JIA compared to controls (Huber and Ward 2016), but comparable bone mineral density in children with JIA versus typically developing children has also been reported (Sandstedt et al. 2012).

The side effects following long-term and high-dose systemic corticosteroids therapy include Cushing syndrome (weight gain, particularly around the midsection and in the face) and possible osteoporosis (Huber and Ward 2016), but since the introduction of biological DMARDs few children with JIA are in need of such treatment.

How to Evaluate the Body Composition of People With JIA

LABORATORY TESTS

Dual-energy X-ray absorptiometry has in recent years been mostly used to measure bone mineral density, and it is also increasingly being used to measure body composition in laboratory and research settings. Bioelectrical impedance analysis has also been used to estimate body composition in JIA. See Chapter 2 for more information about the measurement methods.

FIELD TESTS

Calculating BMI may be the most relevant field test in clinical practice to measure body composition in JIA. Also, as a measure of central body composition, one can assess waist circumference with a measuring tape.

There are no accurate field tests to measure bone mineral density in JIA (or typically developing children).

Effects of Physical Activity on Body Composition in JIA

Even if there is limited evidence on the effect of physical activity on body composition or bone mineral density in JIA, physical activity is considered important to optimize the development of bone mineral density during childhood and adolescence, and to maintain a healthy body composition. Adhering to the recommendations for physical activity for children, including performing physical activities that strengthen muscles and bones, will help to develop normal bone mineral density in JIA. Weight-bearing activities are particularly relevant to ensure normal bone mineral density, but using skeletal muscles is also important to stimulate the development of bone mineral density (World Health Organization 2011).

FLEXIBILITY

Children with JIA may have limited range of motion in joints due to arthritis. A limited range of motion may be present in a single joint or multiple joints depending on the disease severity and JIA category. Swollen joints are usually held in a flexed position. Range of motion may be difficult to evaluate and interpret, as there is a wide range of normal range of motion measurements in children (Kuchta and Davidson 2008). In unilateral involvement with arthritis, it is easier to compare to the joint(s) in the unaffected side. Both the spine and temporomandibular joints (jaw) may be affected.

There is little evidence on the prevalence and severity of limited range of motion in joints in children with JIA after the introduction of biological DMARDs, but clinically there seem to be fewer severe cases of limited range of motion compared to the pre-biological

DMARDs era. Limited range of motion in joint(s) is mostly present at diagnosis and during disease flare-ups.

How to Evaluate the Flexibility of People With JIA

LABORATORY TESTS

Laboratory tests to measure flexibility are not commonly used in JIA.

FIELD TESTS

Flexibility in JIA is measured by range of motion in affected joints by visual estimation or with goniometer in clinical settings. Both active and passive range of motion may be measured. Flexibility may also be evaluated by observation of the child's movement during different activities (e.g. walking, squatting, climbing, and crawling in clinical settings).

Effects of Physical Activity on Flexibility in JIA

There is limited evidence on the effect of physical activity on flexibility in JIA. Yet, when children of JIA have limited range of motion in a joint, they are often recommended to do stretching exercises themselves, with guidance from caregivers if needed. Often there is a need for specific treatment, often physiotherapy and in some cases occupational therapy, to improve range of motion in joints. Treatment of limited range of motion in joints often includes strengthening exercises for muscles near the joint with limited range of motion. There is limited evidence of the effectiveness of these interventions, but clinical experience indicates that most joints with limited range of motion regain normal range of motion.

PROMOTING A PHYSICALLY ACTIVE LIFESTYLE IN YOUNG PEOPLE WITH JIA

The recommendations regarding physical activity and exercise have changed dramatically during the last two decades, often referred to as a paradigm shift. Previously, there were several restrictions regarding physical activity for children with JIA. Contact sports and activities with high intensities were not recommended, while swimming, bicycling using easier gears, and play-acting were recommended activities. These restrictions were applied due to the common well-intentioned belief that physical activity with weight-bearing and high-intensity activities could cause disease flare-ups. Then, based on scientific evidence documenting that exercise was safe in JIA and also beneficial for several outcomes (Klepper 2003), clinical expert experiences, and patients' experiences, children with JIA are now encouraged to participate in physical activities in line with their typically developing peers. There are no general restrictions regarding physical activity for children with JIA. However, precautions may apply for some children in certain cases, and will be discussed later in this chapter. In line with this paradigm shift regarding physical activity in JIA, the physical activity recommendations for children in general are applied in children with JIA as well (see Chapter 5).

In a recent study, vigorous physical activity was identified as a correlate for both higher cardiorespiratory fitness and muscle fitness in children with JIA. In addition to the overall recommendation of performing 60 minutes of moderate-to-vigorous physical activity daily, these results underscore the importance of performing vigorous physical activity and muscle- and bone-strengthening three times per week according to recommendations from health authorities to optimize the health benefits of physical activity in children with JIA (Risum et al. 2018).

Some children with JIA may have difficulties fulfilling these recommendations in periods with high disease activity, and may need adaptations of activities or specific interventions by physiotherapists to target specific impairments (e.g. decreased range of motion in joints subsequent to arthritis). Some children with JIA who have been physically inactive for a prolonged period may need guidance from health care professionals prior to starting exercising by themselves or with peers. Even if the physical activity recommendations are not completely fulfilled, all kinds of physical activity may increase the health benefits from physical activity compared to being sedentary.

Many studies have reported that children with JIA are less physically active and spend more time sedentary compared to controls (Bohr et al. 2015; Norgaard et al. 2016). However, more recent studies have found comparable physical activity levels between children with JIA and controls, possibly explained by improvements in multidisciplinary management in JIA, including biological DMARDs and encouragement to be physically active and participate in activities with peers (Risum et al. 2018, Sherman et al. 2018). The evidence of associations between physical activity levels and disease-related factors is conflicting: associations have been reported between physical activity levels and higher disease activity, arthritis in weight-bearing joints and joint pain, while other studies found no such associations (Bohr et al. 2015; Norgaard et al. 2016; Risum et al. 2018).

A recent study found that children with JIA participated in similar organized and unorganized physical activities as typically developing peers, and that the most reported organized physical activities in both groups of children were dancing and football. Further, the most reported unorganized physical activities in both children with JIA and typically developing peers were jogging/running and strength exercises (Risum et al. 2018). Other studies have reported a lower proportion of children with JIA participating in organized physical activities compared to typically developing controls, and in less intensive activities (Norgaard et al. 2019). Importantly, enjoyment has been highlighted as the most reported facilitator of physical activity in children with JIA and typically developing children (Risum et al. 2018; Norgaard et al. 2019).

School-aged children are advised to participate in physical education at school. Research has shown that an increasing percentage of children with JIA participate in physical education, but that some children may need adaptations of activities to be able to participate (Risum et al. 2018). Different school regulations regarding possibilities for adaptations may vary across countries. Regardless, if a child with JIA has difficulties participating in physical education, cooperation between the child, caregivers, teachers, and health care professionals may enable participation in physical education classes for children with JIA.

Benefits of a Physically Active Lifestyle in JIA

Children with JIA will have the same positive effects of a physical active lifestyle as described for the general population (see Chapter 2). Additionally, physical activity may address and improve several of the symptoms and impairments caused by the disease itself, and further may prevent possible future comorbidities of the disease.

Exercise therapy has been studied in children with JIA using a variety of methods and interventions. Exercise therapies are beneficial across clinically relevant outcomes in JIA (improved functional capacity, knee strength, and quality of life, and decreased pain) (Klepper et al. 2019). However, substantial heterogeneity in exercise interventions and study outcomes has limited the ability to generalize the evidence, and the quality of the exercise studies was evaluated as poor. Importantly, exercise therapy appears to be well tolerated with no adverse effects of exercise reported and exercise therapy does not exacerbate arthritis (Klepper et al. 2019).

Theoretically, a possible anti-inflammatory effect of exercise and physical activity has been proposed in rheumatic diseases, including JIA. New insights into the complex network of immune cells and inflammatory signalling molecules suggest that exercise may contribute to reduce inflammation in rheumatic diseases by the same mechanisms as the biological DMARDs. The use of skeletal muscle produces signalling molecules that are involved in the inflammatory process, yet the exact possible anti-inflammatory effect mechanism is still unknown (Perandini et al. 2012). In adults with inflammatory rheumatic disease, exercise reduced the disease activity significantly (Sveaas et al. 2020).

A physically active lifestyle may also prevent a possible risk of cardiovascular disease in JIA. Furthermore, even if it not well studied, there are reasons to believe that a physically active lifestyle may also prevent an unhealthy body composition (excessive fat mass), which is important in JIA because fat tissue produces pro-inflammatory signalling molecules (Li et al. 2017), with possible negative impact on the disease activity.

Additionally, as mentioned earlier, exercise is important in JIA to improve muscle strength and bone health in children with JIA, in whom muscle strength and bone mineral density often are low compared to typically developing children.

Specific Challenges in JIA

Pain has been addressed as a barrier to being physically active in children with JIA (Risum et al. 2018). Further, fatigue may also be a challenge for some children with JIA. Importantly, physical activity and exercise may improve pain and fatigue in JIA (Klepper et al. 2019). To quantify the intensity of pain and fatigue in JIA, the visual analogue scale or numeric rating scale are widely used measurements. See more on pain and fatigue in Chapter 3.

It is also common for typically developing children to experience episodes of pain and fatigue during childhood and adolescence. Thus, pain and fatigue in children with JIA may not necessarily be symptoms of disease activity.

Some children with JIA experience pain or fatigue even if their JIA is well treated and there are no clinical signs of disease activity of their JIA. When children with JIA experience such persistent pain or fatigue without signs of arthritis or disease activity, it may be helpful to evaluate if other factors may contribute to the experience of pain and fatigue using a biopsychosocial model in the management of pain and fatigue. In more severe cases of pain and fatigue, it can be relevant to involve a multidisciplinary team (e.g. including physiotherapist, paediatric or school nurse, psychologist, occupation therapist, and physician), to help the child and family to cope with pain or fatigue. Physical activity is also important in children with JIA who experience persistent pain or fatigue, as being physically active may reduce pain and fatigue in addition to contributing to health benefits from a physically active lifestyle. It may be easier to perform enjoyable activities when experiencing persistent pain and fatigue. Further, physical activities of shorter duration and lower intensity could also be important for these children, at least if the child has been unable to participate in physical activities for a longer period.

In children with JIA with severe morning stiffness, physical education should preferably take place at the end of the school day.

Specific Recommendations Concerning Involvement of JIA in Certain Joints

Many children with JIA experience few or no challenges to participating in physical activities, while many others may experience challenges requiring some adaptations of physical activities for shorter periods (e.g. disease flare-ups). A few children may experience more severe challenges with being physically active. The following section provides some suggestions for activities related to having arthritis at different body sites.

Having arthritis in the *feet* may cause difficulties participating in weight-bearing activities. Even if the evidence of custom-made foot-orthosis or insoles is scarce, children with JIA may experience pain reduction using them. Covering of costs of these devices may vary across countries. Further, using shoes with shock-absorbing soles is advisable when during physical activities or exercising.

If the arthritis is in the *lower extremities (legs)*, using shoes with shock-absorbing soles is advisable when performing activities like jogging and running. If it is still difficult to perform jogging and running, bicycling and swimming are physical activities that put less load on the joints.

Preschoolers and young school-age children with arthritis in the *hands or wrists* may benefit from playing with clay and finger painting to improve range of motion and grip strength. Older children may find it useful to wear a prefabricated wrist orthosis during physical activities, particularly if the hands are affected, during different ball sports. Using lighter balls may also enable participation, at least in non-competitive activities.

Having arthritis in *several joints* may challenge participation in competitive physical activities. Whenever possible, taking short pauses and lowering the intensity may enable the child with JIA to participate.

In the case of young people with high disease activity with *multiple joints* affected, it may still be possible to perform bicycling, swimming, and strength exercises.

Some Precautions

As in typically developing children, children with JIA should not exercise when they have a fever or infections (see Chapter 3 for general safety considerations).

If a child with JIA experiences increased joint swelling and prolonged joint pain after physical activities or exercise, the treating physician should be contacted to evaluate a possible disease flare-up.

In cases of high disease activity, heart or lung involvement, or use of high doses of systemic corticosteroids or long-term use of systemic corticosteroids, the treating physician should be consulted before a child with JIA starts exercising or engages in physical activity.

REFERENCES

Bohr AH, Fuhlbrigge RC, Pedersen FK, de Ferranti SD, Muller K (2016) Premature subclinical atherosclerosis in children and young adults with juvenile idiopathic arthritis: a review considering preventive measures. *Pediatr Rheumatol Online J* 4: 3.

Bohr AH, Nielsen S, Muller K, Karup Pedersen F, Andersen LB (2015) Reduced physical activity in children and adolescents with juvenile idiopathic arthritis despite satisfactory control of inflammation. *Pediatr Rheumatol Online J* 13: 57.

Cavallo S, Majnemer A, Duffy CM, Feldman DE (2015) Participation in leisure activities by children and adolescents with juvenile idiopathic arthritis. *J Rheumatol* 42: 1708–1715.

Giancane G, Alongi A, Ravelli A (2017) Update on the pathogenesis and treatment of juvenile idiopathic arthritis. *Curr Opin Rheumatol* 29: 523–529.

Houttu N, Kalliomaki M, Gronlund MM, Niinikoski H, Nermes M, Laitinen K (2020) Body composition in children with chronic inflammatory diseases: a systematic review. *Clin Nutr* **39**: 2647–2662.

Huber AM, Ward LM (2016) The impact of underlying disease on fracture risk and bone mineral density in children with rheumatic disorders: a review of current literature. *Semin Arthritis Rheum* **46**: 49–63.

Klepper S, Mano Khan TT, Klotz R, Gregorek AO, Chan YC, Sawade S (2019) Effects of structured exercise training in children and adolescents with juvenile idiopathic arthritis. *Pediatr Phys Ther* **31**: 3–21.

Klepper SE (2003) Exercise and fitness in children with arthritis: evidence of benefits for exercise and physical activity. *Arthritis Rheum* **49**: 435–443.

Kuchta G, Davidson I (2008) *Occupational and Physical Therapy for Children with Rheumatic Diseases: A Clinical Handbook*. Oxford: Radcliffe Publishing.

Lelieveld OT, Takken T, van der Net J, van Weert E (2005) Validity of the 6-minute walking test in juvenile idiopathic arthritis. *Arthritis Rheum* **53**: 304–307.

Li F, Li Y, Duan Y, Hu CA, Tang Y, Yin Y (2017) Myokines and adipokines: involvement in the crosstalk between skeletal muscle and adipose tissue. *Cytokine Growth Factor Rev* **33**: 73–82.

Lindehammar H (2003) Hand strength in juvenile chronic arthritis: a two-year follow-up. *Acta Paediatr* **92**: 1291–1296.

Lindehammar H, Lindvall B (2004) Muscle involvement in juvenile idiopathic arthritis. *Rheumatology* **43**: 1546–1554.

Maggio AB, Hofer MF, Martin XE, Marchand LM, Beghetti M, Farpour-Lambert NJ (2010) Reduced physical activity level and cardiorespiratory fitness in children with chronic diseases. *Eur J Pediatr* **169**: 1187–1193.

Norgaard M, Herlin T (2019) Specific sports habits, leisure-time physical activity, and school-educational physical activity in children with juvenile idiopathic arthritis: patterns and barriers. *Arthritis Care Res* **71**: 271–280.

Norgaard M, Twilt M, Andersen LB, Herlin T (2016) Accelerometry-based monitoring of daily physical activity in children with juvenile idiopathic arthritis. *Scand J Rheumatol* **45**: 179–187.

Perandini LA, de Sa-Pinto AL, Roschel H et al. (2012) Exercise as a therapeutic tool to counteract inflammation and clinical symptoms in autoimmune rheumatic diseases. *Autoimmunity Reviews* **12**: 218–224.

Petty RE, Southwood TR, Manners P et al. (2004) International League of Associations for Rheumatology classification of juvenile idiopathic arthritis: second revision, Edmonton, 2001. *J Rheumatol* **31**: 390–392.

Prakken B, Albani S, Martini A (2011) Juvenile idiopathic arthritis. *Lancet* **377**: 2138–2149.

Rigante D, Bosco A, Esposito S (2015) The etiology of juvenile idiopathic arthritis. *Clin Rev Allergy Immunol* **49**: 253–261.

Ringold S, Angeles-Han ST, Beukelman T et al. (2019) American College of Rheumatology/Arthritis Foundation guideline for the treatment of juvenile idiopathic arthritis: therapeutic approaches for non-systemic polyarthritis, sacroiliitis, and enthesitis. *Arthritis & Rheumatology* **71**: 846–863.

Ringold S, Weiss PF, Beukelman T et al. (2013) Update of the 2011 American College of Rheumatology recommendations for the treatment of juvenile idiopathic arthritis: recommendations for the medical therapy of children with systemic juvenile idiopathic arthritis and tuberculosis screening among children receiving biologic medications. *Arthritis Rheum* **65**: 2499–2512.

Risum K, Edvardsen E, Godang K et al. (2019) Physical fitness in patients with oligoarticular and polyarticular juvenile idiopathic arthritis diagnosed in the era of biologics: a controlled cross-sectional study. *Arthritis Care Res* **71**: 1611–1620.

Risum K, Hansen BH, Selvaag AM, Molberg O, Dagfinrud H, Sanner H (2018) Physical activity in patients with oligo- and polyarticular juvenile idiopathic arthritis diagnosed in the era of biologics: a controlled cross-sectional study. *Pediatr Rheumatol Online J* **16**: 64.

Saarinen J, Lehtonen K, Malkia E, Lahdenne P (2008) Lower extremity isometric strength in children with juvenile idiopathic arthritis. *Clin Exp Rheumatol* **26**: 947–953.

Sandstedt E, Fasth A, Fors H, Beckung E (2012) Bone health in children and adolescents with juvenile idiopathic arthritis and the influence of short-term physical exercise. *Pediatr Phys Ther* **24**: 155–161.

Sherman G, Nemet D, Moshe V et al. (2018) Disease activity, overweight, physical activity and screen time in a cohort of patients with juvenile idiopathic arthritis. *Clin Exp AQ Volumer Rheumatol* **36**: 1110–1116.

Shoop-Worrall SJW, Kearsley-Fleet L, Thomson W, Verstappen SMM, Hyrich KL (2017) How common is remission in juvenile idiopathic arthritis: a systematic review. *Semin Arthritis Rheum* **47**: 331–337.

Sveaas SH, Bilberg A, Berg IJ et al. (2020) High intensity exercise for 3 months reduces disease activity in axial spondyloarthritis (axSpA): a multicentre randomised trial of 100 patients. *Br J Sports Med* **54**: 292–297.

van Pelt PA, Takken T, van Brussel M, de Witte I, Kruize AA, Wulffraat NM (2012) Aerobic capacity and disease activity in children, adolescents and young adults with juvenile idiopathic arthritis (JIA). *Pediatr Rheumatol Online J* **10**: 27.

World Health Organization (2011) *Global Recommendations on Physical Activity for Health 5–17 Years Old*. Geneva: World Health Organization.

Index